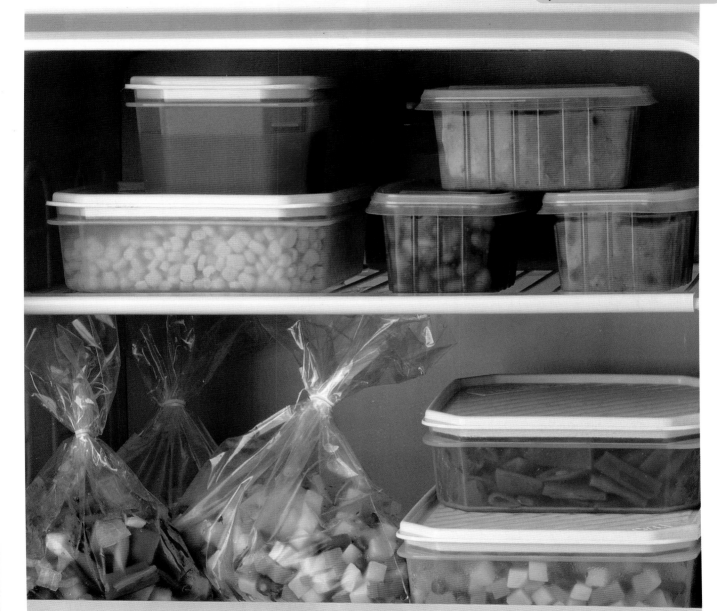

Text © 2011 Michele Borboa, M.S.
Photography and Design © 2011 Fair Winds Press

First published in the USA in 2011 by:
Fair Winds Press, a member of
Quayside Publishing Group
100 Cummings Center
Suite 406-L
Beverly, MA 01915-6101
www.fairwindspress.com

15 14 13 12 11          2 3 4 5

ISBN-13: 978-1-59233-463-6
ISBN-10: 1-59233-463-6
Digital edition published in 2011
eISBN-13: 978-1-61058-060-1

Library of Congress Cataloging-in-Publication Data available

Cover and book design by Carol Holtz | holtzdesign.com
All photography by Bill Bettencourt with the exception of the following:
© foodanddrinkphotos/agefotostock.com, 59
© FoodCollection/agefotostock.com, 41
© Hrbkova\Sporrer/agefotostock.com, 81
© Mirko Iannace/agefotostock.com, 147
iStockphoto.com, 1; 7; 10; 12; 15; 21; 99; 125; 163; 203
© Tetra Images/agefotostock.com, 179

Printed and bound in China

# MAKE-AHEAD MEALS MADE HEALTHY

**EXCEPTIONALLY DELICIOUS AND NUTRITIOUS FREEZER-FRIENDLY RECIPES
YOU CAN PREPARE IN ADVANCE AND ENJOY AT A MOMENT'S NOTICE**

## MICHELE BORBOA, M.S.

# CONTENTS

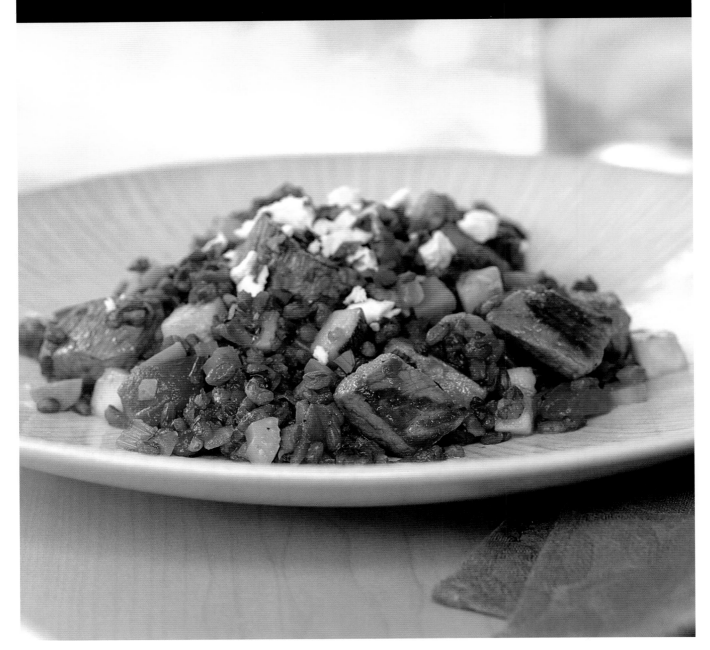

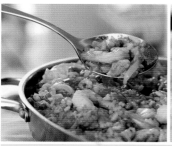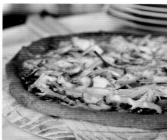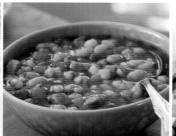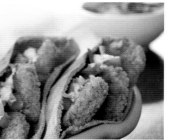

# CHAPTER 1

# GETTING STARTED
## ALL YOU NEED TO KNOW FOR FANTASTIC FREEZER-FRIENDLY MEALS

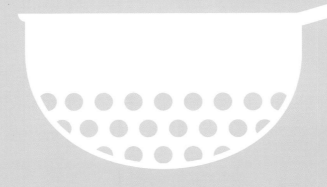

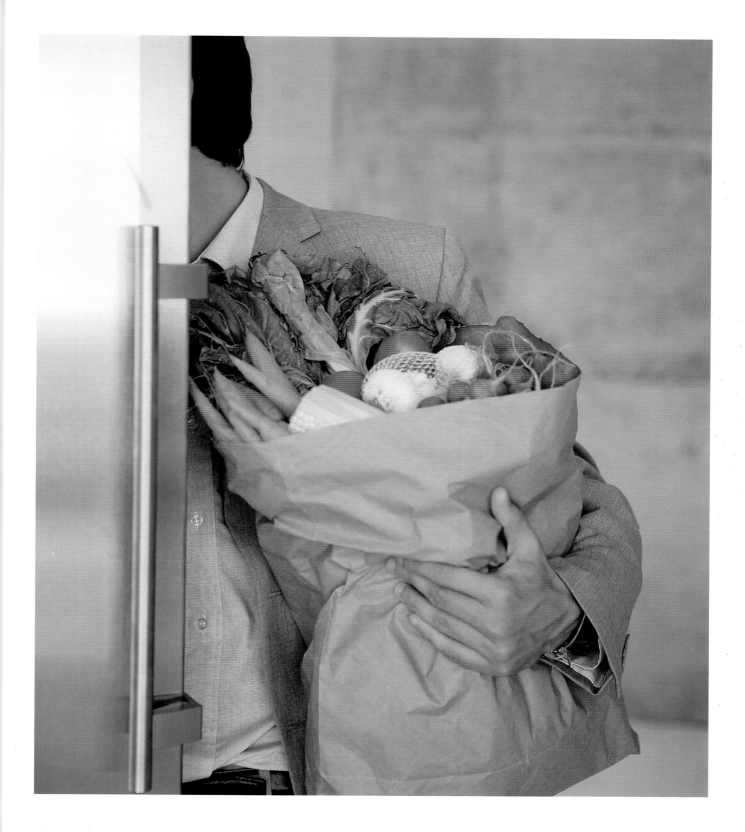

IN TODAY'S BUSY WORLD, families sitting down at the table for home-cooked meals is a rarity. Frequently, meals are eaten at restaurants—or too often from the drive-thru—or from meals pulled from the supermarket freezer section and reheated in the microwave. The result of too many meals out and overconsumption of processed, packaged foods is families who are overweight; a growing number of children suffering from chronic weight-related diseases, such as type 2 diabetes; and a disconnect of families from the enjoyment of sit-down meals made (even mostly) from scratch.

Eating out, dining by delivery, drive-thrus, and grocery store frozen main courses not only put your health and waistline at risk, but they are expensive and in many cases, take just as much time, if not more, than cooking a meal at home. Gathering your family around the kitchen dinner table or even better, having the family help with the meal before it gets to the dinner table, is a tasty opportunity to spend quality time together. Best yet, by making meals at home, you are teaching your kids a valuable lesson in health-promoting, money-saving life skills. Your kids will grow up with the perspective that home-cooked meals are the norm—even for the busiest of families.

So how do you accomplish healthfully feeding your family every day without spending most of your day slaving in the kitchen? By learning the art of make-ahead meals! Fixing and freezing meals is an easy, cost-effective, and long-term solution to keeping your family well-fed at home as well as on-the-go.

As you page through this book, you'll find recipes ranging from eye-opening breakfasts and comfort food casseroles to succulent meats and lip-smacking sweets—all of which can be frozen and reheated effortlessly, yielding meals that are not just as tasty as meals made on the spot, but even better, given the time they've been given (in the freezer) for their flavors to mingle and develop.

In addition to recipes for all tastes and occasions, you'll find guidelines for successfully fixing and freezing meals, both for individual servings and for feeding a crowd, as well as detailed reheating and serving suggestions for every single recipe.

Make-ahead meals do require some time up front, but the result is a future of delicious, stress-free meals that can be put on the table in a manner of minutes. Ready to get cooking?

# FIX-AND-FREEZE 101

Fixing and freezing your own selection of ready-to-heat eats is a simple and easy process to master, no matter what your level of "freezing expertise." Here is all you need to know to get started— in just nine easy steps!

### Step #1: Stay Well-Stocked

Keeping your kitchen stocked with essential ingredients will help ensure you can put together a healthy meal—whether it is make-ahead or not—without having to run to the store. Staple ingredients are nutritious, packed with flavor, and endlessly versatile.

**TEN STAPLES FOR THE HEALTHY MAKE-AHEAD KITCHEN**

#### 1. Canned Beans

A stellar source of protein, fiber, and other health-promoting nutrients, canned beans are one of the most versatile ingredients in the kitchen. They have a long shelf life and as an ingredient in make-ahead recipes, do well in the freezer.

#### 2. Frozen Fruits and Vegetables

A daily trip to the supermarket for fresh produce isn't feasible for most busy families. Keeping a variety of frozen fruits and vegetables on hand not only gives you a convenient way to include nutrient-rich produce in your weekly meals, it also keeps a ready supply of healthy ingredients to add to your fix-and-freeze feasts. Some of my favorite frozen fruits and vegetables to keep on hand include: blueberries, marionberries, mango, sliced bananas (you can easily package these yourself), peas, corn, edamame, lima beans, and mixed vegetables.

#### 3. Dry Pasta, Rice, and Other Grains and Flours

The palate-pleasing plethora of whole-grain pastas, rice, and other grains such as quinoa, millet, and barley give you a near endless array of wholesome

## TASTY AND CREATIVE USES FOR CANNED BEANS

Puréed for dips, such as hummus ● Used as a thickener for sauces ● Tossed into salads for a meat-free protein alternative ● Simmered in soups, stews, and chili ● Added to burrito and enchilada fillings ● Used as a base for vegetarian burgers

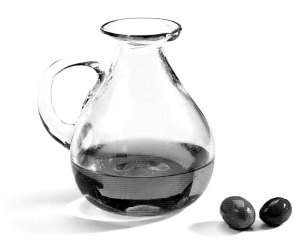

make-ahead possibilities. These staples can be cooked ahead and frozen as is or included in recipes before freezing (see Family-Favorite Freezer Rice, page 110).

Opt for high-fiber pastas, whole-wheat couscous, brown or wild rice, and the many whole grains you can find in the bulk section of your local natural food stores or in the grain aisle at the supermarket. In addition, keep a bag each of whole-wheat pastry flour and all-purpose flour for baking, breading, and thickening.

### 4. Olive or Canola Oil

No kitchen pantry should be without at least one heart-healthy cooking oil. Both olive and canola oils are rich in good-for-you monounsaturated fats and can be used for a variety of culinary applications. Because of its delicate nature, extra-virgin olive oil should only be used for salad dressings or to drizzle on cooked foods, while pure olive oil can withstand higher heat cooking, such as sautéing. Canola oil has

a very mild flavor, which is ideal for many baked goods, and can also be used in higher-heat cooking.

### 5. Eggs

Eggs are a tasty go-to for breakfast and brunch, necessary for baking, and, when hard cooked, can quickly become the base for egg-salad sandwiches or added to macaroni salad, potato salad, and tuna salad. Hard-cooked eggs can also be tossed with green salads or vegetables. Eggs come in handy when making fix-and-freeze quiche, bread pudding, quick breads, cakes, cookies, and even ice cream.

Though eggs are perishable, they do have a good shelf life if stored properly in the refrigerator. Do not store eggs in the refrigerator door since it is opened often and subject to temperature fluctuations.

### 6. Cheese

Dry, grating cheeses such as Parmesan and Romano are loaded with flavor (so a little goes a long way), hugely versatile, and have a long shelf life. They will last in the fridge six months unopened and three to four months opened.

Key in lasagna and other pasta dishes, these Italian cheeses are also essential ingredients for pesto and even savory breads. For the best flavor, buy a wedge and grate the amount you need for your recipe on the spot. The same goes for blocks of semi-firm cheese, such as Cheddar and Swiss, which are also easy to keep on hand and can be quickly shredded into recipes.

Other, softer cheeses such as feta and blue cheese make good staples too. They don't have the shelf life of dry cheeses, but their distinctive characteristics will give your make-ahead meals a delectable punch of flavor.

### 7.  Onions, Garlic, and Other Flavorful Ingredients

Onions and garlic are frequently used in savory recipes, laying the flavor foundation for meat dishes, stir-fries, sauces, and more. Keep in mind that the shelf life of onions and garlic will widely vary depending on when they were harvested or purchased. If stored properly, however, most store-bought onions will stay fresh for three weeks or longer, while whole heads of garlic will last one month or longer (the shelf life of garlic decreases once the cloves are separated). Be sure to choose onions and heads of garlic that are firm, unblemished, and show no signs of mold and keep them stored in a cool, dark place so they are within easy reach when you start to cook.

Dried herbs and spices are one of the most convenient ways to add fabulous flavor to all of your meals. There is no need to buy every available herb and spice; simply stock your spice rack with these tasty essentials: Italian seasoning, 5-spice powder, chili powder, curry powder, cinnamon, cumin, coriander, nutmeg, paprika, rosemary, sage, and other dried herbs and spices you know you will use. The bare minimum is salt (try a good sea salt) and black peppercorns, which you can freshly grind upon need.

In addition to keeping dried herbs and spices on hand, if you have the room, grow your own fresh herbs. They add great flavor to savory recipes and even desserts, such as the Decadent Dark Chocolate Mint Cake (page 208). Whether you're new to growing herbs or a seasoned gardener, the best herbs to grow are the ones that you'll use. My basic fresh herb arsenal includes rosemary (which is very hardy), flat-leaf parsley (a great overall flavor enhancer),

 **COOKING TIP: FREEZING FRESH GINGER**

Fresh ginger is an unparalleled ingredient with a distinctive flavor that dried ginger does not provide. Though the knobby root can last up to one month in your refrigerator wrapped in plastic wrap, keeping a ready supply in your freezer means you'll always have ginger root within reach.

To freeze fresh ginger: Peel ginger and slice crosswise into $1/8$-inch (3 mm) coins. Place coins on a plate or baking sheet in one layer; freeze until solid. Store frozen ginger coins in a freezer bag.

To use ginger: Thaw frozen ginger slightly, and then mince and add to your recipe. Mincing while still semifrozen makes it an easier and neater job.

cilantro (ideal for giving food fresh Mexican flair), chives (perfect for potatoes, chicken, fish, and dressings), and basil (cinnamon and Thai basils are my favorite).

Fresh ginger is another flavorful ingredient to keep in the refrigerator or freezer. Store fresh ginger in a paper bag in the refrigerator or see "Freezing Fresh Ginger" (page 11).

### 8. Sun-Dried Tomatoes Packed in Olive Oil

Meaty and packed with flavor, sun-dried tomatoes add rich color and fantastic flavor to just about any meal. They can be puréed into pesto, dressings, and sauces, added to sautéed meat and vegetable dishes, tossed with salads, or even incorporated into delicious savory quick bread and scone recipes. Dry-packed tomatoes can be rehydrated with hot water (and are usually less expensive), but buying sun-dried tomatoes in olive oil deliciously saves you a prep step.

### 9. Low-Sodium Broth

A tasty alternative to plain water when cooking rice and other grains, broth can also be used to deglaze meats and vegetables, add flavor to soups and stews, and transform sauces. Low-sodium vegetable, chicken, and beef broths are especially heart-healthy

choices because they add their characteristic flavors while allowing you to season your dishes according to your tastes. Broths are conveniently available in cans and aseptic boxes. Be sure to read the labels and avoid broths containing MSG or gluten for family members with food sensitivities. For shelf-life dates, check the label on the container.

### 10. Lean Meats, Skinless Poultry, Seafood, and Other Lean Protein

A ready-source of protein and the centerpiece for many family meals, meat, poultry, and seafood can be bought fresh from your reputable local butcher right before you launch into your make-ahead meal making, or you can keep a variety in your freezer. To defrost, simply place meat, poultry, or seafood in the refrigerator to thaw the day before you plan to cook. If you are vegetarian, keep shelf-stable boxes of tofu (made by Mori-Nu) in your pantry or refrigerator. Keep track of the expiration dates on the boxes and use them before they expire.

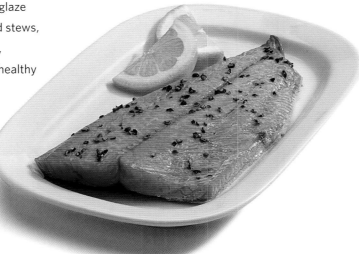

## Step #2: Pick Out Your Recipes

Before you head to the supermarket with make-ahead meals in mind, sit down and make a list of the recipes you want to make. Whether you want to fix and freeze meals for the next week or for the next two months, you need a list of the ingredients necessary to prepare them. Check your pantry, refrigerator, and freezer first to see if you already have ingredients on hand and then determine the ingredients you have to purchase. To further save you time and money and reduce the risk of waste, make recipes that share similar ingredients.

## Step #3: Schedule Your Make-Ahead Meal Making

Make sure you schedule your cooking time closely after your food shopping to maximize nutrients from fruits and vegetables as well as prepare food at its freshest. The amount of time you need is dependent on the dishes—and number of dishes—you've decided to make. Set aside a Sunday afternoon or early evening during the week, or if you are an early bird, start cooking after your first cup of coffee (bonus: the kitchen is cooler in the morning!).

## Step #4: Get Organized

Arrange your ingredients in the order you will use them and set your cookware, measuring tools, and utensils on the counter for easy access. Go through your freezer and discard any foods that have freezer burn, have been sitting in there since last year, or that you won't eventually consume (if you're concerned about wasting food, give them to a neighbor or someone else who might find them useful). Arrange the remaining freezer items so you have room to store your soon-to-come freezer-friendly meals.

## Step #5: Prep Your Ingredients

The last thing you want to do while cooking a dish is realize you need to finely chop two large onions, skin the chicken thighs, or defrost the berries. Before you launch into your meal prepping, read the recipes and

### SAFETY FIRST!

When cooking, always make sure to do the following: • Keep raw meat, poultry, and fish away from grains, produce, and other food. • Use separate cutting boards for raw meats/poultry/seafood and produce. • Wash your hands before and right after handling raw foods. • Place prepped perishable foods in the refrigerator until ready to use if you aren't immediately using them. • Sharpen your knives. Dull knives are often more dangerous than sharp ones because it requires more force to cut with a dull knife, which increases the risk of losing control of it and cutting yourself.

prep ingredients accordingly. Use a variety of bowls to hold ingredients for each recipe; for example, if a recipe calls for sautéing diced onions, carrots, and celery, place them all in a bowl and add them to the pot when the oil is hot.

## Step #6: Get Cooking!

Now that you have your cookware and ingredients in place, it's time to get cooking. When cooking multiple meals, consider starting with the most time-intensive recipes (i.e., a yeast bread that takes 50 minutes to rise or a stew that simmers for an hour). You can use the downtime to prepare other dishes. Recipes that require a slow cooker can be started the night before or in the morning. The amount of time you spend on cooking these make-ahead meals may seem intensive now, but remember, you are making meals—perhaps double and triple batches of recipes—that will conveniently feed your family for days and weeks to come.

## Step #7: Cool Cooked Foods Completely

After you've cooked your meals, let them cool at room temperature for no more than two hours and then refrigerate until completely cool. This minimizes the risk of bacteria growth and it will ensure your make-ahead meals freeze better. Freezing foods only once completely cooled not only better preserves their taste and texture, but also reduces the risk of moisture becoming trapped in the container, bag, or wrap and creating freezer burn.

Here are some other cooling tips:

- If you're in a hurry, divide large batches into smaller portions; smaller portions cool faster.
- Place food in freezer bags and lay flat; flat thin items cool faster than thick ones. Just be sure to avoid placing hot food items in the bags, as the plastic could melt.
- Do not stack containers or bags of hot or warm foods on top of one another; arrange them side by side to cool quicker (with lids left off, or ajar if possible).

## Step #8: Freeze Smartly

Taking the time to properly package and store your meals will deliver great-tasting dishes, while also guaranteeing efficient use of your freezer space. Here are a few handy tips to keep in mind for making your dishes as freezer-friendly as possible.

### FREEZING TIP #1: USE THE RIGHT SUPPLIES

Having and using the right freezer supplies will help optimize your freezer space while also freeing up your baking dishes. Following is a list of the items I find most essential and how to use each most efficiently.

### Freezer Bags

Pour cooled sauces, soups, stews, and chili into heavy-duty freezer bags and seal. Lay them on their side in a baking dish, stacking multiple bags, and freeze. Once solid, take them out of the baking dish and stack in freezer (vertically or horizontally—

whatever saves the most space). To thaw, set bag in a baking dish and place in the refrigerator.

### Plastic Freezer Paper or Wrap

Self-sealing freezer paper or wrap can be used in place of foil and freezer bags for many dishes. To use, line an empty baking dish with a piece of freezer wrap large enough to cover the bottom, sides, and over the top of the dish. Transfer a cooked, completely cooled meal to the baking dish, seal the freezer wrap, and freeze. When food is solid, remove it from the baking dish and stack in the freezer. To thaw, remove freezer wrap, place frozen food in baking dish, cover with foil, and refrigerate.

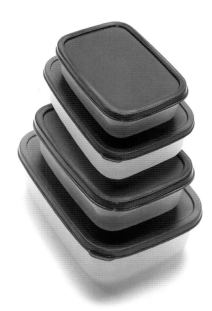

### Aluminum Foil

If you don't want to freeze foods in your usual bakeware or don't have aluminum bakeware, aluminum foil can come to your rescue. Before you place a recipe in a baking dish, line the dish with heavy-duty aluminum foil. Prepare dish according to recipe directions. After cooling completely, cover dish with foil and place in freezer until solid. Lift frozen food from the baking dish and tightly wrap with a second layer of heavy-duty foil and return to the freezer. Stack subsequent frozen foods. To thaw, remove foil, put frozen food back in original dish and follow reheating instructions.

### Aluminum Bakeware

Cook recipes in aluminum bakeware according to recipe directions. Once completely cooled, place a layer of plastic wrap right on the food, tightly wrap

with heavy-duty aluminum foil and then freeze. If the bakeware came with a lid, you can put that on top too (assuming you have the space). To thaw, peel back foil, remove plastic wrap, replace foil, and place in refrigerator.

### Freezer and Microwave-Safe Containers

Though individual serving–size containers aren't space efficient, they do offer the convenience of reheating single or smaller portions of fix-and-freeze meals. To optimize space, stack them neatly in the freezer. To thaw, simply put containers in the refrigerator.

### Permanent Markers or Labels

Use markers or adhesive labels, whichever you prefer. We'll cover labeling specifics in tip #3.

## FREEZING TIP #2: PACKAGE ACCORDING TO SERVINGS NEEDED

Most of the recipes in this book serve eight to ten. When packaging your make-ahead meals for freezing, consider the number of servings you will need when it's time to reheat. You can package recipes, such as Beef, Black Bean, and Mango Enchiladas (page 24) or Meatless Butternut Squash and Chard Lasagna (page 35), in single-serving containers to reheat in the microwave at work or when dining solo at home. You might want to package other recipes in larger batches, like the Elegant and Easy Stuffed Chicken Breasts with Wild Rice (page 65 ) or Venison Black Bean Chili (page 91), so you can serve a crowd. To cover all of your needs, we've provided packaging instructions for both individual and "crowd-size" servings wherever possible.

## FREEZING TIP #3: LABEL WITH DETAIL

Once you package your foods in appropriate freezer-safe wrap or containers, label them. Whether you write directly on a bag or affix adhesive labels, include the date frozen, name of the dish, serving size, reheating instructions and if needed, additional ingredients, such as guacamole for burritos, chopped veggies or crumbled cheese to garnish a soup, or a side of rice for a stir-fry. In addition, be sure to make a list of dishes in your freezer so you are always aware of your make-ahead inventory.

### PACKAGING FOR LONGEVITY

Though foods can be frozen much longer than they can be refrigerated, you still want to package them in the most efficient way to maximize their life span in the freezer. Ensure quality by doing the following: • Make sure your freezer temperature is between −5°F (−21°C) and 0°F (−18°C). • Let food cool completely before packaging. • Use heavy-duty freezer bags instead of plastic storage bags. • Use heavy-duty aluminum foil instead of lightweight foil. • Remove as much air as possible from bags and containers before sealing. • Double-bag meats, poultry, or seafood that contains bones to prevent leakage in the case bones puncture the bag. • Freeze individual items, such as muffins, scones, waffles, chicken strips, and meatballs on baking sheets until solid, then transfer to freezer bags, remove as much air as possible, seal bag, and place back in the freezer. • Keep older meals in the front of the freezer so they are eaten in a timely manner.

**FREEZING TIP #4: HEED SHELF-LIFE DATES**

Though some foods may be fine longer in the freezer, the following shelf-life estimates are provided for yielding the best results when reheating or after thawing. Try to serve your meals and food items well before their dates are up to ensure the best flavor and taste.

# HOW LONG IS IT GOOD FOR?

| Food | | Freezer Shelf Life |
|---|---|---|
| Fruits and Vegetables | Frozen fresh fruit | 8 to 12 months |
| | Fruit frozen with syrup or sugar | 12 months |
| | Freezer jams | 12 months |
| | Frozen fresh vegetables | Up to 1 year |
| | Tomato sauce | 6 months |
| Breakfast Items | Waffles and pancakes | 2 months |
| | Scones and muffins | 2 months |
| | Quick breads | 2 months |
| | Quiche | 2 months |
| Yeast Breads and Pizza | Breads, rolls, soft pretzels | 2 to 3 months |
| | Unbaked bread dough | 2 months |
| | Pizza dough | 2 months |
| | Baked pizza crust (with or without toppings) | 2 months |
| | Focaccia | 2 months |
| | Bread crumbs | 2 to 3 months |
| Casseroles | Poultry casseroles | 4 months |
| | Meat casseroles | 4 months |
| | Baked pasta | 2 to 3 months |

# HOW LONG IS IT GOOD FOR? (continued)

| Food | | Freezer Shelf Life | |
|---|---|---|---|
| **Meats, Poultry, and Seafood** | Ground meat or poultry | 3 to 4 months | |
| | Uncooked burger patties | 3 to 4 months | |
| | Cooked burger patties | 2 to 3 months | |
| | Uncooked lamb, pork, beef steaks, and chops | 6 months | |
| | Cooked lamb, pork, beef steaks, and chops | 2 months | |
| | Uncooked lamb, pork, and beef roasts | 4 to 6 months | |
| | Bacon, sausage, and hot dogs | 1 to 2 months | |
| | Uncooked chicken or turkey | 6 months | |
| | Cooked chicken or turkey | 2 to 3 months | |
| | Cooked chicken strips | 2 months | |
| | Deli meats | 1 to 2 months | |
| | Uncooked fish | 3 to 6 months | |
| | Cooked fish | 2 months | |
| | Uncooked shellfish | 3 to 6 months | |
| | Cooked shellfish | 2 months | |
| **Soups, Stews, and Chili** | Chili | 4 to 6 months | |
| | Broth-based soups | 4 to 6 months | |
| | Stews | 4 to 6 months | |
| | Stock or broth | 3 to 4 months | |
| **Grains** | Cooked rice | 2 to 3 months | |
| | Cooked quinoa, millet, and other grains | 2 to 3 months | |
| | Cooked pasta | 2 to 3 months | |

# HOW LONG IS IT GOOD FOR? (continued)

| Food | | Freezer Shelf Life |
|---|---|---|
| **Dairy** | Butter | 6 to 9 months |
| | Soft cheese (texture will change) | 2 to 3 months |
| | Firm cheese (texture will change) | 3 to 4 months |
| | Cream and half-and-half | 2 months |
| | Milk (texture will change, best for cooking) | 1 month |
| | Sour cream (texture will change, best for cooking) | 2 months |
| **Desserts** | Cookie dough | 6 months |
| | Baked cookies | 4 to 6 months |
| | Pie dough | 3 months |
| | Ready-to-bake pie crust | 2 months |
| | Baked fruit pies | Up to 1 year |
| | Unbaked fruit pies | 6 to 8 months |
| | Pumpkin pie | 1 to 2 months |
| | Layer cakes (unfrosted) | 2 to 3 months |
| | Cheesecakes | 4 to 6 months |
| | Sponge cakes and angel food cakes | 2 to 3 months |
| | Coffee cakes | 2 to 3 months |
| | Homemade ice cream | 2 to 4 months |

## Step #9: Thaw, Reheat, and Eat!

Most recipes in this book call for thawing frozen dishes in the refrigerator, though some recipes, such as breads, can be thawed directly on the counter. We provide specific reheating instructions in each recipe, so as to ensure both the quality and deliciousness of your meals. Happy eating!

**Final note:** For those recipes where a range of servings is provided, nutritional analysis is based on the larger number of servings.

# CHAPTER 2

# CASEROLES
## THE QUINTESSENTIAL FIX-AND-FREEZE DISH

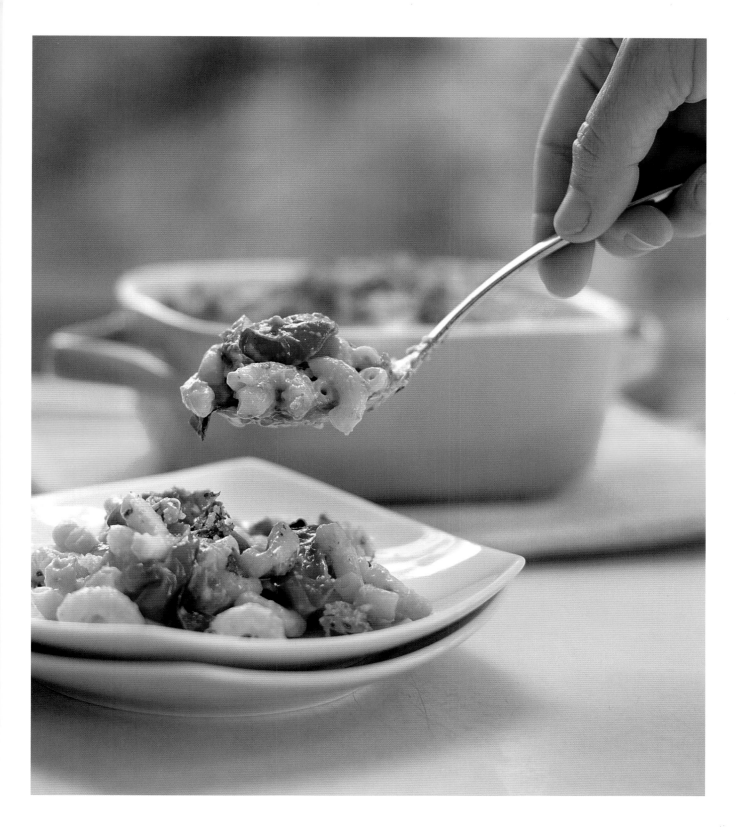

# POTLUCK-PERFECT TAMALE PIE

A one-dish meal, the combination of ground beef, vegetables, and corn bread will quickly become a weeknight family favorite. This Mexican-inspired dish is also ideal for potlucks and spectator-sport parties.

........................................................................................................................................

2 tablespoons (28 ml) olive oil

½ onion, chopped

Salt and freshly ground black pepper

1 teaspoon cumin

1 teaspoon coriander

1 teaspoon dried oregano

2 cloves garlic, minced

¾ pound (340 g) extra-lean ground beef

2 tablespoons (12 g) grated lime zest

2 scallions, chopped

1 can (15 ounces, or 425 g) diced tomatoes

1 can (4 ounces, or 115 g) diced green chiles

1 cup (140 g) sliced black olives

3 cups (700 ml) water

1 cup (140 g) coarse cornmeal

1 teaspoon paprika

1 cup (154 g) corn kernels

¾ cup (86 g) shredded Mexican blend cheese

① Preheat oven to 350°F (180°C, or gas mark 4). Spray a 11 x 7-inch (28 x 18 cm) baking dish with cooking spray and set aside.

② Heat olive oil in a large skillet over medium-high heat. Add onion and a little salt and pepper. Cook, stirring often, until onions are softened. Stir in cumin, coriander, oregano, and garlic, cooking for 1 minute.

③ Add beef and cook, stirring often, until browned. Stir in lime zest and scallions, cooking for 1 minute. Add tomatoes, chiles, and olives, stirring to combine. Cook until heat through. Reduce heat to low.

④ Meanwhile, bring water to a boil in a medium saucepan. Add cornmeal and season with salt and pepper. Whisk continually until mixture starts to thicken. Add paprika and corn and continue to whisk until cornmeal has a thick oatmeal consistency. Stir in cheese. Remove from heat.

⑤ Spoon beef mixture into prepared baking dish, spreading evenly. Pour cornmeal mixture over top and spread evenly to cover.

⑥ Bake for 30 minutes or until corn bread topping is set. Cool completely on a wire rack.

YIELD: 8 SERVINGS

 ## TO FREEZE

INDIVIDUAL SERVINGS: Place individual portions into freezer- and microwave-safe containers and freeze.

FOR A CROWD: Place a layer of plastic wrap directly on top of the corn bread topping. Tightly cover dish in heavy-duty aluminum foil.

 ## TO REHEAT

Thaw in refrigerator overnight.

MICROWAVE METHOD: Reheat individual servings in the microwave at 60% power for 3 minutes or until heated through.

OVEN METHOD: Preheat oven to 350°F (180°C, or gas mark 4). Remove foil and plastic from baking dish. Re-cover dish with foil and bake for 30 minutes or until heated through.

AMOUNT PER SERVING: Calories 266.14; Total Fat 10.31 g; Cholesterol 33.25 mg; Sodium 277.18 mg; Potassium 683.96 mg; Total Carbohydrates 30.61 g; Fiber 7.42 g; Sugar 8.53 g; Protein 15.89 g

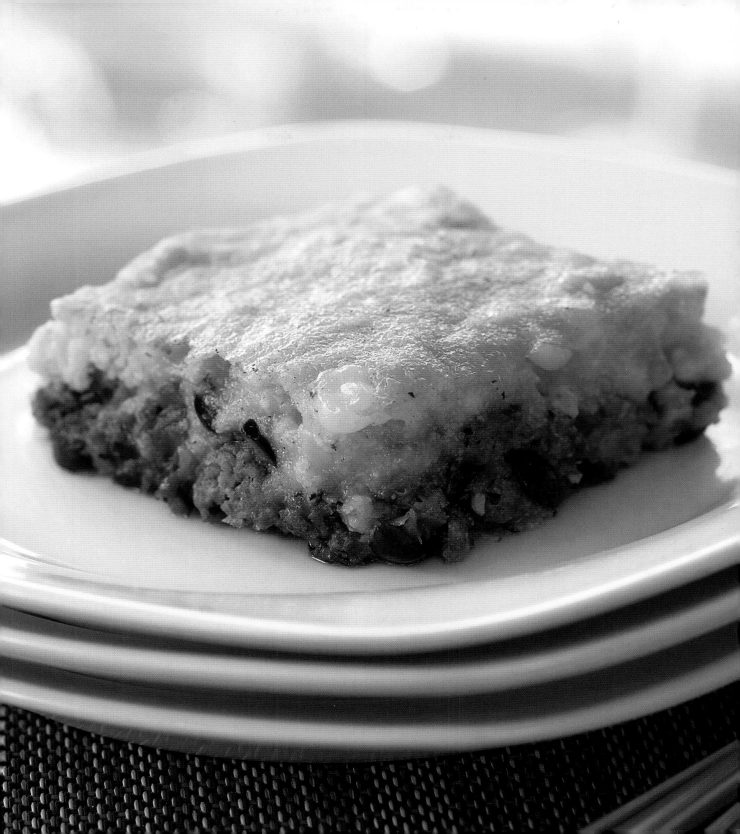

# BEEF, BLACK BEAN, AND MANGO ENCHILADAS

Beef and black beans meet sweet mango in these inventive enchiladas, bursting with antioxidants, protein, and fiber. For a tasty change, substitute lean ground turkey for the beef, papaya for the mango, and cilantro for the mint.

1 tablespoon (15 ml) olive oil

1 pound (455 g) extra-lean ground beef

1 teaspoon smoked paprika

1 teaspoon ground cumin

1 teaspoon ground coriander

salt to taste

Freshly ground black pepper to taste

Grated zest and juice of 1 lime

1 bunch scallions, ends trimmed, chopped (green and white parts)

1 very ripe mango, pitted, peeled, chopped

1 can (15 ounces, or 425 g) black beans, rinsed, drained

3 tablespoons (18 g) finely chopped fresh mint

½ cup (115 g) sour cream

¾ cup (113 g) crumbled feta cheese, divided

1 can (28 ounces, or 785 g) red enchilada sauce

8 (8-inch, or 20 cm) whole-grain flour tortillas

① Preheat oven to 350°F (180°C, or gas mark 4) and generously spray an 11 x 7-inch (28 x 18 cm) baking pan with cooking spray.

② Heat oil in a Dutch oven over medium-high heat. Add beef and cook, stirring often to break it up, for 3 minutes. Sprinkle with paprika, cumin, coriander, salt, black pepper, and lime zest and juice. Cook, stirring, until beef is no longer pink.

③ Reduce heat to medium. Add onions and mango and cook, stirring occasionally, for 2 to 3 minutes. Stir in the black beans and chopped mint and cook, stirring occasionally, for 2 to 3 minutes. Stir in sour cream and ½ cup (75 g) feta and remove from heat.

④ Heat enchilada sauce in a wide skillet over low heat. Dip a tortilla in sauce, coating both sides, and allow excess sauce to drip off. Place tortilla in the baking pan and fill with beef mixture. Roll filling in tortilla and arrange tortilla seam-side down against the side of the baking pan.

⑤ Repeat with remaining tortillas and beef mixture. Pour remaining sauce over enchiladas and sprinkle with remaining feta.

⑥ Cover pan with foil and bake for 20 minutes. Remove foil and bake for an additional 10 minutes. Let cool completely.

YIELD: 8 SERVINGS

 TO FREEZE

INDIVIDUAL SERVINGS: Place individual enchiladas in freezer- and microwave-safe containers.

FOR A CROWD: Tightly cover baking pan with heavy-duty aluminum foil.

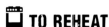 TO REHEAT

Let enchiladas thaw in the refrigerator overnight.

MICROWAVE METHOD: Reheat individual enchiladas in the microwave on high for 2 to 3 minutes or until heated through.

OVEN METHOD: Preheat oven to 350°F (180°C, or gas mark 4). Keep pan covered with foil and bake for 20 minutes.

AMOUNT PER SERVING: Calories 413.14; Total Fat 16.4 g; Cholesterol 55.7 mg; Sodium 558.57 mg; Potassium 858.61 mg; Total Carbohydrates 45.97 g; Fiber 9.6 g; Sugar 5 g; Protein 23.5 g

# LEAN, MEAN MEXICAN TURKEY AND RICE CASSEROLE

*Try*

This is a Mexican-inspired casserole that is reminiscent of stuffed peppers but baked in a dish. Spicy ground turkey stands in for beef while brown rice replaces the white rice typically found in stuffed pepper recipes.

3 tablespoons (45 ml) olive oil, divided

2 pounds (900 g) lean ground turkey

Salt and freshly ground black pepper

2 tablespoons (18 g) chipotle pepper in adobo sauce, finely chopped

2 teaspoons dried oregano

1 onion, finely chopped

2 poblano peppers, seeded, cut into thin strips

2 red bell peppers, seeded, cut into thin strips

2 cloves garlic, minced

2 cans (14.5 ounces, or 410 g, each) fire-roasted diced tomatoes or 4 cups (720 g) Fire-Roasted Tomatoes (page 39)

1 teaspoon ground coriander

1 teaspoon ground cumin

½ teaspoon paprika

3 cups (585 g) cooked brown rice

1 cup (154 g) fresh corn kernels

¼ cup (4 g) finely chopped fresh cilantro

1½ cups (173 g) crumbled Manchego cheese

① Heat 1 tablespoon (15 ml) olive oil in a large pot over medium-high heat. Add turkey, salt and pepper, chipotle, and oregano and cook, stirring often, until turkey is browned. Remove from pot and set aside.

② Add remaining oil to pot and cook onion and peppers, stirring often, until vegetables are softened and lightly browned. Season with salt and pepper. Add garlic and cook, stirring often, for 1 minute. Add tomatoes, coriander, cumin, and paprika and bring to a boil. Reduce heat to low and simmer for 5 minutes. Stir in turkey, rice, corn, and cilantro. Let cool completely. Stir in Manchego cheese.

YIELD: 8 SERVINGS

## SERVING SUGGESTION

A crisp and colorful salad is the perfect accompaniment for this hearty bake. Toss together grapefruit segments, red onion, shredded romaine, pumpkin seeds, and diced avocado with a drizzle of olive oil and fresh lemon juice.

 ## TO FREEZE

INDIVIDUAL SERVINGS: Divide turkey and rice mixture among 8 freezer- and microwave-safe containers.

FOR A CROWD: Transfer turkey and rice mixture to a greased 13 x 9-inch (33 x 23 cm) baking dish. Cover with freezer wrap or plastic and aluminum foil.

 ## TO REHEAT

Let turkey and rice mixture thaw in refrigerator overnight.

MICROWAVE METHOD: Individual servings can be reheated in the microwave on high for 2 minutes or until heated through.

OVEN METHOD: Preheat oven to 350°F (180°C, or gas mark 4). Remove freezer wrap or plastic from baking dish. Cover with aluminum foil and bake for 20 minutes. Remove foil and bake for 10 more minutes or until heated through.

AMOUNT PER SERVING: Calories 520.87; Total Fat 25.86 g; Cholesterol 89.59 mg; Sodium 225.06 mg; Potassium 1018.81 mg; Total Carbohydrates 38.73 g; Fiber 7.82 g; Sugar 8.6 g; Protein 31.26 g

# FAST-FIX CHICKEN AND VEGGIE ENCHILADAS

My mom's chicken enchiladas are still a tasty, healthy hit. I've added mushrooms and spinach to boost nutrition and cut calories, red and green enchilada sauce to keep them intriguing, and whole-wheat flour tortillas for extra fiber.

**1 pound (455 g) boneless, skinless chicken breast, diced small**

**Salt and freshly ground black pepper to taste**

**1 tablespoon (15 ml) olive oil**

**1 cup (70 g) sliced mushrooms**

**1 clove garlic, minced**

**Zest, minced and juice of 1 lemon**

**1 teaspoon ground cumin**

**1 teaspoon ground coriander**

**3 cups (90 g) baby spinach, washed**

**4 scallions, diced (green and white parts)**

**1 can (7 ounces, or 198 g) diced green chiles**

**½ cup (115 g) light sour cream**

**2 cups (230 g) shredded Monterey Jack cheese, divided**

**1 can (28 ounces, or 785 g) green enchilada sauce**

**8 (10-inch, or 25 cm) whole-wheat flour tortillas**

**Whole black olives**

**Chopped fresh cilantro**

① Season chicken with salt and pepper. Heat oil in a large skillet over medium heat. Add chicken and cook for 3 minutes, stirring often, to brown.

② Add mushrooms and cook, stirring often, for 2 minutes. Cover and let cook until mushrooms start to soften. Add garlic, lemon zest and juice, spices, and spinach. Stir thoroughly. Cover with lid and cook until spinach starts to wilt. Stir well and check chicken for doneness; it should be cooked through.

③ Transfer chicken mixture to a large mixing bowl. Add scallions, sour cream, and 1 cup (115 g) Monterey Jack cheese, stirring to combine. Set aside. (Filling can be made to this point and refrigerated up to 2 days.)

④ Preheat oven to 375°F (190°C, or gas mark 5). Spray an 11 x 7-inch (28 x 18 cm) baking dish with nonstick cooking spray and set dish by the stovetop. Pour enchilada sauce into a large skillet over medium-low heat.

⑤ When sauce is warm, dip both sides of a tortilla into sauce, allowing excess to drip off. Place tortilla against the short side of the baking dish and fill with chicken mixture. Roll tortilla around filling, tucking in the edges and arranging it seam-side down. Repeat with remaining tortillas and filling.

⑥ Pour remaining warm sauce over enchiladas. Sprinkle with remaining cheese. Spray a large piece of foil with nonstick cooking spray and use it to cover baking dish with the sprayed side down (this will keep the cheese from sticking to it).

⑦ Bake for 20 to 25 minutes or until sauce is bubbling. Remove foil and cook 10 more minutes to lightly brown cheese. Remove from oven and let cool.

YIELD: 8 SERVINGS

 **TO FREEZE**

INDIVIDUAL SERVINGS: Freeze individual enchiladas in freezer- and microwave-safe containers.

FOR A CROWD: Tightly wrap baking dish with freezer wrap.

**TO REHEAT**

Let enchiladas thaw completely in refrigerator overnight.

MICROWAVE METHOD: Reheat individual servings in microwave on high for 2 to 3 minutes or until heated through. Serve with olives and cilantro.

OVEN METHOD: Preheat oven to 350°F (180°C, or gas mark 4). Remove freezer wrap and cover dish with aluminum foil. Bake for 20 minutes or until heated through. Serve with olives and cilantro.

AMOUNT PER SERVING: Calories 445.35; Total Fat 18.34 g; Cholesterol 65.2 mg; Sodium 1246.45 mg; Potassium 726.63 mg; Total Carbohydrates 40.72 g; Fiber 16.42 g; Sugar 14.53 g; Protein 31.62 g

# LIGHTENED-UP MAC AND CHEESE

Mac and cheese gets a healthy update with the addition of whole-wheat penne pasta and frozen spinach. Sharp Cheddar, Gouda, and cottage cheese are unparalleled stand-ins for the artificial orange-colored goop from a box. For a change, stir in chopped Roasted Red Peppers (page 139), sun-dried tomatoes, and fresh herbs.

⅓ cup (37 g) dry whole-wheat bread crumbs or Whole-Grain Bread Crumbs (page 175)

2 tablespoons (28 ml) olive oil

1 package (16 ounces, or 455 g) frozen spinach

3½ cups (820 ml) milk, divided

6 tablespoons (48 g) all-purpose flour

2 cups (225 g) shredded extra-sharp Cheddar cheese

2 cups (240 g) shredded Gouda cheese

2 cups (450 g) low-fat cottage cheese

½ teaspoon freshly grated nutmeg

Salt and freshly ground black pepper to taste

1 pound (455 g) whole-wheat penne

½ teaspoon freshly grated nutmeg

① Generously spray a 13 x 9-inch (33 x 23 cm) baking dish or aluminum pan with cooking spray. Bring a large pot of salted water to boil.

② In a small bowl, toss together bread crumbs and olive oil. Cook spinach according to package directions. Drain and refresh under cold water. Press out excess moisture. Set aside.

③ In a large saucepan over medium-high heat, bring 3 cups (700 ml) milk to a low simmer. In a small bowl, whisk together remaining milk and flour until smooth. Whisk flour mixture into the hot milk mixture, whisking constantly, until sauce thickens.

④ Remove saucepan from heat and stir in Cheddar and Gouda, stirring until cheese melts. Stir in cottage cheese and season with nutmeg, salt, and pepper.

⑤ Cook pasta in the pot of boiling water for 3 minutes less than package directions, about 6 minutes. Drain in a colander and add to cheese sauce, stirring to combine.

⑥ Spread half of the pasta mixture in the prepared baking dish. Spoon spinach over top. Top with remaining pasta and sprinkle with bread crumbs. Let dish cool completely or refrigerate overnight.

YIELD: 10 SERVINGS

 ## TO FREEZE

INDIVIDUAL SERVINGS: Divide mac and cheese among 10 freezer- and microwave-safe dishes.

FOR A CROWD: Generously spray a sheet of plastic wrap with cooking spray and lay on top of the mac and cheese. Tightly wrap with heavy-duty aluminum foil.

 ## TO REHEAT

Let mac and cheese thaw in the refrigerator overnight.

MICROWAVE METHOD: Individual portions can be reheated in the microwave on high for 2 to 3 minutes or until heated through.

OVEN METHOD: Preheat oven to 400°F (200°C, or gas mark 6). Remove foil and plastic from baking dish. Bake for 30 minutes or until heated through and bubbly.

AMOUNT PER SERVING: Calories 416.69; Total Fat 20.68 g; Cholesterol 71.67 mg; Sodium 180.05 mg; Potassium 865.45 mg; Total Carbohydrates 30.98 g; Fiber 6.25 g; Sugar 6.88 g; Protein 25.00g

# WHOLE-GRAIN PESTO PASTA CASSEROLE

Turkey sausage is a lower-fat substitute for pork varieties, giving this scrumptious baked pasta dish a healthy edge over other renditions.

1 tablespoon (15 ml) olive oil

1 onion, chopped

3 cloves garlic, minced

1 pound (455 g) spicy Italian turkey sausage, casings removed, crumbled

1 can (28 ounces, or 795 g) fire-roasted diced tomatoes, drained, or 3¾ cups (675 g) Fire-Roasted Tomatoes (page 39)

½ cup (120 ml) red wine

pinch of salt

Freshly ground black pepper to taste

¾ cup (195 g) store-bought pesto or Toasted Almond and Basil Pesto (page 169)

1 pound (455 g) whole-wheat medium-size pasta shells

1¾ cups (193 g) shredded fontina cheese

¼ cup (25 g) grated Parmesan cheese

① Preheat oven to 400°F (200°C, or gas mark 6). Spray a 13 x 9-inch (33 x 23 cm) baking dish or aluminum pan with cooking spray. Bring a large pot of salted water to a boil.

② Heat oil in a Dutch oven over medium heat. Add onion and cook, stirring often, until onion is softened. Add garlic and cook, stirring, for 1 minute. Add sausage and cook, stirring occasionally, until sausage is browned.

③ Stir in tomatoes, wine, salt, and pepper. Bring to a simmer and allow to cook for 5 to 6 minutes or until almost all of the liquid evaporates. Stir in pesto and remove from heat.

④ Cook pasta in boiling water for 2 to 3 minutes less than package directions, about 7 minutes. Drain in a colander. Toss pasta with sauce.

⑤ Pour half of the pasta mixture into prepared baking dish. Sprinkle with half of the fontina and Parmesan. Pour remaining pasta over top and sprinkle with remaining cheese. Bake for 15 minutes until cheese is melted and bubbly. Set on a wire rack to cool completely.

YIELD: 10 SERVINGS

## SERVING SUGGESTION

Pair this bake with a vegetable dish for a balanced meal. Here are some suggestions:

- Green salad with radicchio, romaine, olives, shaved Parmesan, and sun-dried tomatoes
- Quick and Snappy Beans with Hazelnuts (page 100)
- Roasted asparagus drizzled with olive oil
- Tender Roasted Vegetables (page 105)
- Fast and Fabulous Fava Beans (page 106)
- Sautéed leafy greens with garlic, olive oil, and lemon zest

## TO FREEZE

INDIVIDUAL SERVINGS: Divide pasta into 10 freezer- and microwave-safe dishes and freeze.

FOR A CROWD: Generously spray a sheet of plastic wrap with cooking spray and lay it on top of the pasta. Tightly cover with heavy-duty aluminum foil.

## TO REHEAT

Let pasta thaw in refrigerator overnight.

MICROWAVE METHOD: Reheat individual servings in the microwave on high for 2 to 3 minutes or until heated through.

OVEN METHOD: Preheat oven to 400°F (200°C, or gas mark 6). Remove foil and plastic wrap from the baking dish. Bake in the oven for 20 to 25 minutes or until cheese is melted and pasta is heated through.

AMOUNT PER SERVING: Calories 521.05; Total Fat 26.22 g; Cholesterol 66.01 mg; Sodium 755.81 mg; Potassium 521.30 mg; Total Carbohydrates 47.29 g; Fiber 5.24 g; Sugar 6.44 g; Protein 22.28 g

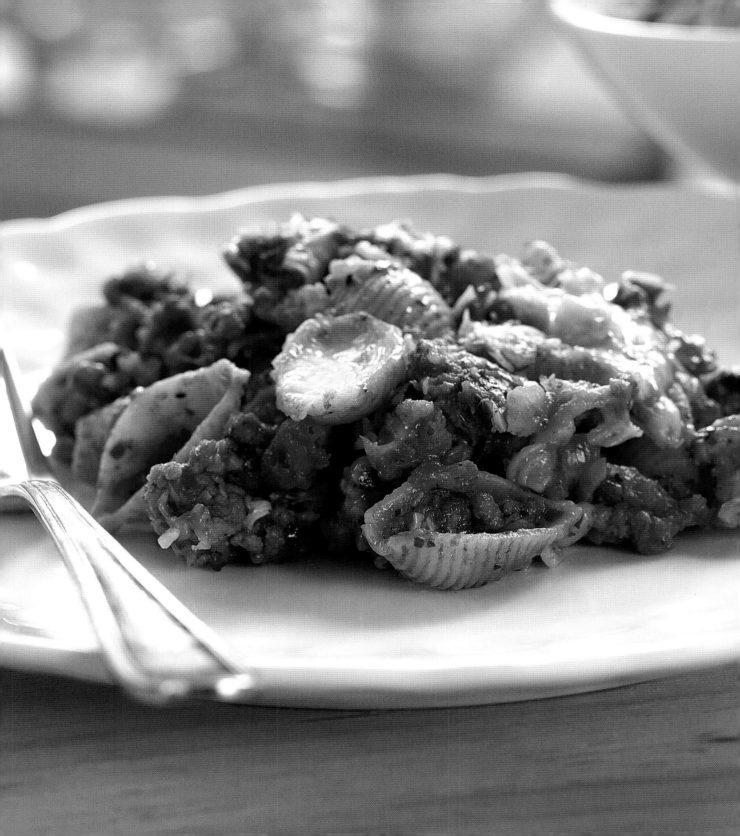

# MUSHROOM-STUFFED PORK CHOPS WITH ROASTED ROOT VEGETABLES

Though not technically a casserole, these juicy stuffed pork chops on a bed of roasted root vegetables is a healthy and hearty one-dish fall or winter meal that comes together in 30 minutes.

FOR THE ROASTED VEGETABLES:

**1 sweet potato, cut into bite-size chunks**

**2 carrots, thickly sliced crosswise**

**1 turnip, cut into bite-size chunks**

**1 bunch radishes, trimmed**

**2 tablespoons (28 ml) olive oil**

**Salt and freshly ground black pepper to taste**

**½ cup (120 ml) vegetable broth**

FOR THE PORK CHOPS:

**8 boneless center-cut pork loin chops**

**Salt and freshly ground black pepper to taste**

**3 tablespoons (45 ml) olive oil, divided**

**1 tablespoon (14 g) unsalted butter**

**4 slices whole-wheat bread, cubed**

**½ onion, diced**

**1 large stalk celery, finely chopped**

**8 ounces (225 g) sliced wild mushrooms, such as cremini, shiitake, oyster, or morel**

**1 clove garlic, minced**

**⅓ cup (37 g) finely chopped sun-dried tomatoes packed in olive oil**

**1 tablespoon (2 g) minced fresh rosemary**

**1 cup (320 g) apricot preserves**

**Juice of 1 lemon**

①  Preheat oven 400°F (200°C, or gas mark 6). Toss vegetables in olive oil and season with salt and pepper. Set them in a roasting pan and roast, stirring every 4 to 5 minutes, for 20 minutes or until vegetables are tender and lightly browned. Remove from oven, pour in broth, and set aside. Do not turn off oven.

②  Slice a pocket in the side of each pork chop. Season inside and out with salt and pepper. Set aside. In a large skillet over medium heat, heat 1 tablespoon (15 ml) olive oil and butter, swirling pan to melt butter. Add bread cubes and cook, stirring often, until bread is lightly toasted. Transfer bread to a plate.

③  In the same skillet, add 1 tablespoon (15 ml) olive oil and heat to medium. Add onion and celery and cook, stirring often, for 3 minutes. Add mushrooms and garlic and cook for 3 minutes. Add sun-dried tomatoes and rosemary and cook, stirring often, for 3 to 4 minutes. Season with salt and pepper.

④  Add bread cubes to skillet and toss to combine. Stuff pork chops with mushroom mixture and set aside. Heat remaining oil in skillet over medium-high heat. In batches, brown pork chops, cooking each side for 2 to 3 minutes.

⑤  Place pork chops in a greased 13 x 9-inch (33 x 23 cm) baking dish and place in the oven uncovered. Cook for 5 minutes or until pork is just cooked through. Remove from oven. In a small bowl, whisk together apricot preserves and lemon juice. Microwave on high for 30 seconds and drizzle over pork chops.

⑥  Cool for 30 minutes and then refrigerate until completely cool.

YIELD: 8 SERVINGS

 **TO FREEZE**

INDIVIDUAL SERVINGS: Divide vegetables and pork chops among 8 freezer- and microwave-safe containers.

FOR A CROWD: Arrange vegetables around pork chops in baking dish. Cover tightly with freezer wrap or wrap with plastic then aluminum foil.

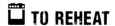 **TO REHEAT**

Let pork chops and vegetables thaw in refrigerator overnight.

MICROWAVE METHOD: Individual servings of pork chops and vegetables can be reheated in the microwave on 60% power for 2 to 3 minutes or until heated through. Don't overcook pork or it will be dry.

OVEN METHOD: Preheat oven to 375°F (190°C, or gas mark 5). Remove freezer wrap or plastic from baking dish and cover with aluminum foil. Bake for 30 minutes or until heated through.

AMOUNT PER SERVING: Calories 596.12; Total Fat 18.09 g; Cholesterol 126.07 mg; Sodium 339.91 mg; Potassium 1558.99 mg; Total Carbohydrates 65.32 g; Fiber 7.39 g; Sugar 21.98 g; Protein 47.95 g

# CREAMY TURKEY CASSEROLE WITH BROCCOLI AND CAULIFLOWER

Cancer-fighting cruciferous vegetables meet lean, mean turkey breast for a healthy casserole that comes together in mere minutes. For a change, substitute broccoli and cauliflower for other vegetables you happen to have on hand.

**3 cups (213 g) broccoli florets**

**3 cups (300 g) cauliflower florets**

**6 cups (840 g) chopped cooked skinless turkey breast**

**1½ cups (263 g) chopped dried prunes**

**2 cans (10.75 ounces, or 305 ml each) low-fat reduced-sodium cream of chicken soup**

**1 cup (225 g) light mayonnaise made with olive oil**

**1 cup (160 g) finely chopped red onion**

**¼ cup (15 g) finely chopped fresh parsley**

**1 tablespoon (2 g) fresh thyme**

**2 cups (230 g) shredded Havarti cheese, divided**

**Salt and freshly ground black pepper to taste**

① Steam broccoli and cauliflower until fork-tender. Chop coarsely and set aside to cool.

② In a large bowl, combine turkey, prunes, soup, mayonnaise, onion, parsley, thyme, and 1 cup (112 g) Havarti. Stir in broccoli and cauliflower. Season with salt and pepper.

YIELD: 10 SERVINGS

## TO FREEZE

INDIVIDUAL SERVINGS: Divide turkey mixture among 10 freezer- and microwave-safe containers. Sprinkle with remaining Havarti before sealing.

FOR A CROWD: Line a 13 x 9-inch (33 x 23 cm) baking dish with enough freezer wrap to generously cover bottom, overlap side, and fold over top. Transfer turkey mixture to baking dish and sprinkle with remaining cheese. Seal freezer wrap. Freeze until solid and then lift casserole out of dish and stack in freezer.

## TO REHEAT

Let individual servings thaw in refrigerator overnight. For entire casserole, remove freezer wrap and place in original baking dish and thaw overnight.

MICROWAVE METHOD: Reheat individual servings in the microwave on 50% power, stirring every minute, for 3 to 4 minutes or until heated through.

OVEN METHOD: Preheat oven to 375°F (190°C, or gas mark 5). Cover casserole dish with foil and bake for 20 minutes. Remove foil and bake for 10 more minutes or until cheese is melted and lightly browned.

AMOUNT PER SERVING: Calories 416.69; Total Fat 20.68 g; Cholesterol 71.67 mg; Sodium 180.04 mg; Potassium 865.44 mg; Total Carbohydrates 30.98 g; Fiber 6.25 g; Sugar 6.88 g; Protein 25.00g

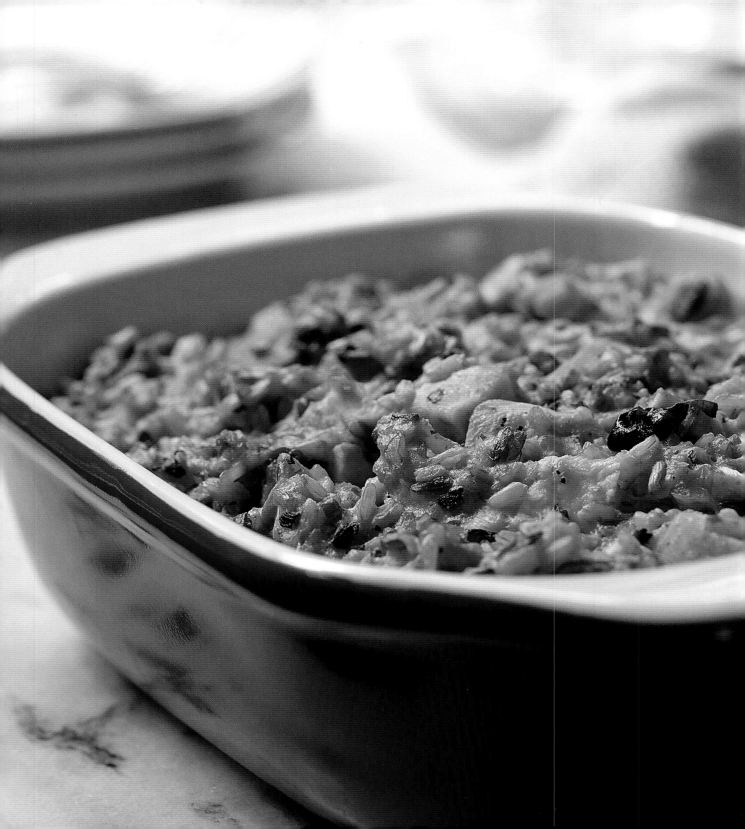

# FAMILY-FRIENDLY CHICKEN AND WILD RICE BAKE

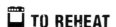

Chicken, wild rice, fresh herbs, and dried fruit make this one-dish dinner a mouthwatering mélange of tastes and textures. A hearty meal for cold autumn and winter days, dividing it into individual serving sizes will give you and your kids a filling lunch to anticipate when you need a meal to beat the chill.

2 cups (320 g) wild rice

4 cups (950 ml) low-sodium chicken broth

2 cups (475 ml) water

1 cup finely chopped dried fruit, such as cherries (160 g), apricots (130 g), or raisins (145 g)

3 tablespoons (12 g) finely chopped fresh parsley

Juice of 1 small lemon

2 tablespoons (12 g) grated lemon zest

Salt and freshly ground black pepper

3 cups (420 g) chopped cooked skinless chicken breast

1½ cups (150 g) chopped scallions (green and white parts)

1 tablespoon (4 g) finely chopped fresh tarragon leaves

2 cans (10.75 ounces, or 305 ml each) low-fat reduced-sodium cream of chicken soup

1 cup (230 g) light sour cream

 ① In a large pot over high heat, bring rice, broth, and water to a boil. Reduce heat to low, cover pot, and cook rice according to package directions. Stir in dried fruit, parsley, lemon juice, and zest. Spread rice onto a rimmed baking sheet and cool completely.

② In a large bowl, combine rice, chicken, scallions, and tarragon. Add chicken mixture, cream of chicken soup, and sour cream and stir to combine. Season with salt and pepper.

YIELD: 8 SERVINGS

## ▮ TO FREEZE

INDIVIDUAL SERVINGS: Divide chicken and rice mixture among 8 freezer- and microwave-safe containers or 1-quart (950 ml) freezer bags, removing as much air as possible before sealing.

FOR A CROWD: Line a 13 x 9-inch (33 x 23 cm) baking dish with enough freezer wrap to generously cover bottom, overlap the sides, and fold over the top. Pour chicken and rice mixture into baking dish and seal freezer wrap. Freeze until solid and then lift frozen casserole out and stack in freezer.

## ▭ TO REHEAT

Let individual servings of chicken and rice mixture thaw in the refrigerator overnight. For entire casserole, remove freezer wrap, place frozen casserole in original baking dish, and let thaw overnight.

MICROWAVE METHOD: Reheat individual servings in the microwave on 50% power, stirring every minute, for 3 to 4 minutes or until heated through.

OVEN METHOD: Preheat oven to 375°F (190°C, or gas mark 5). Cover baking dish with foil and bake for 20 minutes. Remove foil and bake for 10 minutes more.

### COOKING TIP: SOAK WILD RICE

Wild rice takes longer to cook than conventional rice—soaking the rice for a few hours or even overnight can shorten the cooking time. You can cook wild rice in three ways: boiling, steaming, or absorption. Cooking times will vary, so be sure to keep an eye on it.

AMOUNT PER SERVING: Calories 496.08; Total Fat 9 g; Cholesterol 58.94 mg; Sodium 2006.81 mg; Potassium 1238.56 mg; Total Carbohydrates 77.78 g; Fiber 5.81 g; Sugar 2.93 g; Protein 29.52 g

# SMOKED TROUT AND JASMINE RICE CASSEROLE

A delectable change from smoked salmon, smoked trout gives this casserole a unique flavor and a way to get your daily quota of omega-3 fatty acids. If smoked trout is unavailable, simply swap in your favorite smoked sockeye salmon.

**2 cups (370 g) jasmine rice**

**4 cups (950 ml) low-sodium vegetable broth**

**2 tablespoons (28 ml) olive oil**

**3 carrots, finely chopped**

**2 celery stalks, finely chopped**

**1 onion, finely chopped**

**6 cups (180 g) spinach leaves**

**Salt and freshly ground black pepper to taste**

**1 can (10.75 ounces, or 305 ml) condensed cream of mushroom soup**

**1¾ cups (425 ml) water**

**¼ cup (15 g) finely chopped fresh parsley**

**1½ cups (175 g) shredded Italian blend cheese**

**2½ cups (340 g) flaked smoked trout**

① Preheat oven to 350°F (180°C, or gas mark 4) and grease a 13 x 9-inch (33 x 23 cm) baking dish.

② In a medium saucepan, bring jasmine rice and vegetable broth to a boil. Reduce heat to medium-low and simmer for 15 to 18 minutes or until water is absorbed. Remove from heat.

③ Heat oil in a stockpot over medium heat and add carrots, celery, and onion. Cook, stirring often, until vegetables are just tender. Add spinach, in batches if necessary, and cook, stirring often, until spinach is wilted. Season with salt and pepper.

④ Stir in soup, water, parsley, ¾ cup (86 g) cheese, and trout. Stir in rice. Pour into prepared baking dish and sprinkle with remaining cheese. Bake for 30 minutes. Let cool completely.

YIELD: 8 SERVINGS

## NUTRITION SPOTLIGHT: TROUT

In addition to being inexpensive, trout is a tasty nutritional catch. A 3-ounce (85 g) cooked portion provides around 130 calories, 22 grams of protein, 5 grams of healthy fats, and no carbohydrates. Including trout in your diet can help you meet the heart-healthy recommendation of dining on fish twice per week. If fresh trout doesn't bait your hook, try smoked trout, available at many fish counters and for order online.

##  TO FREEZE

INDIVIDUAL SERVINGS: Divide casserole among 8 freezer- and microwave-safe containers.

FOR A CROWD: Cover baking dish with freezer wrap.

## TO REHEAT

Let casserole thaw in refrigerator overnight.

MICROWAVE METHOD: Individual servings can be reheated in the microwave on 60% power for 2 to 3 minutes or until heated through.

OVEN METHOD: Preheat oven to 350°F (180°C, or gas mark 4). Remove freezer wrap and cover dish with aluminum foil. Bake for 20 minutes. Remove foil and bake 10 more minutes.

AMOUNT PER SERVING: Calories 361.07; Total Fat 14.64 g; Cholesterol 22.16 mg; Sodium 1624.11 mg; Potassium 308.2 mg; Total Carbohydrates 19.14 g; Fiber 1.85 g; Sugar 2.96 g; Protein 21.68 g

# MEATLESS BUTTERNUT SQUASH AND CHARD LASAGNA

Winter squash and chard are filling yet low-calorie stars in this mouthwatering meatless lasagna. Flavorfully rich in color and deliciously laden with vitamins and minerals, your family will never notice it is meat-free.

**1 (2-pound, or 900 g) butternut squash**

**Sea salt and freshly grated black pepper to taste**

**1 tablespoon (15 ml) olive oil, divided**

**2 cloves garlic, minced**

**1 shallot**

**8 ounces (225 g) baby spinach leaves, washed, drained, but left damp**

**1 container (16 ounces, or 455 g) part-skim ricotta**

**½ cup (40 g) shredded Parmesan cheese**

**1 teaspoon dried oregano**

**1 teaspoon freshly grated nutmeg**

**1 teaspoon ground cinnamon**

**1 bunch red chard, washed, drained, but left damp**

**1 jar (28 ounces, or 785 g) spicy marinara sauce**

**8 uncooked whole-wheat lasagna noodles**

**1½ cups (175 g) shredded mozzarella cheese**

① Chop the shallot. Remove stems from chard and coarsely chop.

② With a knife or fork, poke holes or small slits all over squash. Place on a microwave-safe plate and microwave on high for 5 to 6 minutes or until a knife inserts easily into the skin. Microwaving instead of baking the squash saves time and makes it easier to peel.

③ Let squash stand for 5 minutes or until cool enough to handle. Use a vegetable peeler to remove skin. Cut squash in half lengthwise and using a spoon, remove seeds. Slice thinly and season with salt and black pepper. Set aside.

④ Preheat oven to 350°F (180°C, or gas mark 4) and spray a 13 x 9 x 2-inch (33 x 23 x 5 cm) baking dish with nonstick cooking spray.

⑤ In a large nonstick saucepan, heat oil over medium-high heat. Cook garlic and shallot, stirring frequently, until soft, 3 to 4 minutes. Add spinach and cook, stirring, until wilted, 3 to 4 minutes.

⑥ Transfer spinach and any liquid to a medium bowl to cool slightly. Stir in ricotta, Parmesan, oregano, nutmeg, and cinnamon. Set aside.

⑦ In the same saucepan, add chard and season with salt and pepper. Press down and stir with a spatula for 1 to 2 minutes. Cover and cook until wilted, stirring occasionally, and adding a bit more water if pan gets dry, about 5 to 6 minutes. Set aside.

⑧ Pour ½ cup (125 g) marinara into the prepared baking dish, using the back of a spoon to evenly spread. Lay 3 or 4 noodles in sauce. Spread half of the ricotta cheese mixture on noodles. Layer with butternut squash. Lay 3 or 4 noodles on squash and cover with half of the marinara sauce. Cover with chard and spread remaining ricotta cheese mixture on top. Cover with remaining noodles and sauce. Sprinkle with mozzarella.

⑨ Spray a large piece of foil with nonstick cooking spray and use it to tightly cover dish. Bake lasagna until sauce is bubbly, about 50 to 55 minutes. Remove foil and cook for 5 to 10 minutes more to brown cheese. Remove from oven and let stand at least 15 minutes before cutting.

YIELD: 10 SERVINGS

AMOUNT PER SERVING: Calories 433.4; Total Fat 12.99 g; Cholesterol 30.36 mg; Sodium 650.63 mg; Potassium 1041.18 mg; Total Carbohydrates 66.66 g; Fiber 9.98 g; Sugar 9.93 g; Protein 21.2 g

*Recipe continued on next page*

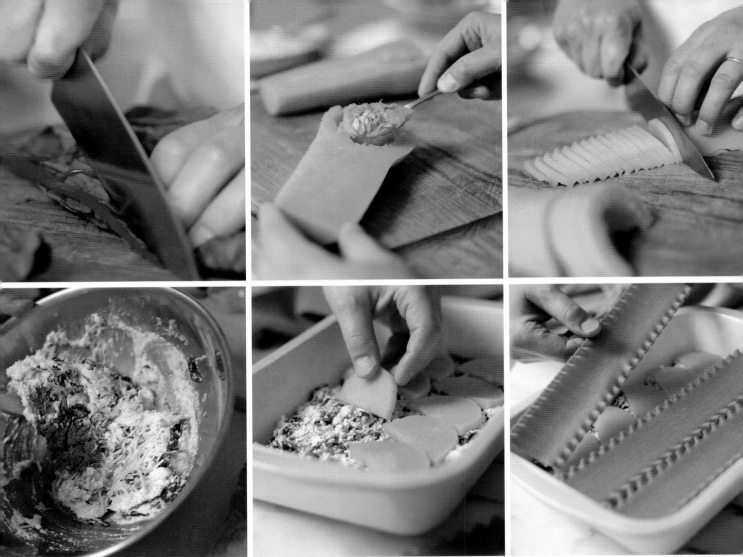

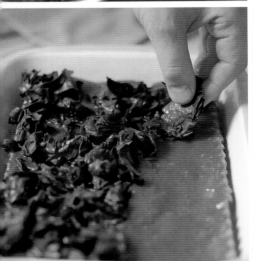

## 🧊 TO FREEZE

INDIVIDUAL SERVINGS: Divide lasagna into 10 freezer- and microwave-safe containers.

FOR A CROWD: Let Lasagna cool completely. Cover with a sheet of plastic wrap placed directly on the lasagna. Cover pan tightly with aluminum foil,

## 🍳 TO REHEAT

Let lasagna thaw in refrigerator overnight.

MICROWAVE METHOD: Individual portions can be reheated in the microwave on high for 2 to 3 minutes or until heated through.

OVEN METHOD: Preheat oven to 375°F (190°C, or gas mark 5). If reheating single portions, place desired number of pieces into baking dish. If reheating entire pan, carefully take foil off of baking dish and remove plastic wrap. Cover baking dish with foil and cook in oven for 35 to 40 minutes or until lasagna is hot and bubbling.

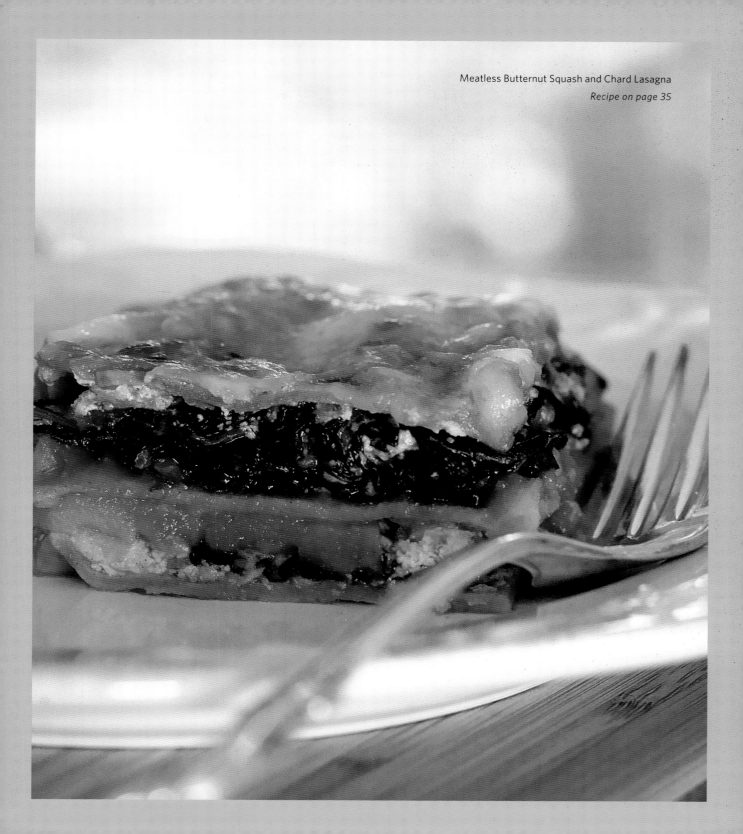

Meatless Butternut Squash and Chard Lasagna
*Recipe on page 35*

# CREAMY MUSHROOM EMPAÑADAS

Traditionally stuffed with meat and cheese, these empañadas are packed with meaty mushrooms and blanketed with a mildly spicy green sauce.

2 pounds (900 g) mix of wild mushrooms, such as shiitake, chanterelles, or porcini

2 tablespoons (28 ml) olive oil

2 cloves garlic, minced

1 teaspoon dried thyme

Pinch of salt

Freshly ground black pepper to taste

3 tablespoons (3 g) finely chopped fresh cilantro

1 cup (230 g) light sour cream

8 ounces (225 g) Neufchâtel cheese, cut into small cubes

1 can (28 ounces, or 785 g) mild green enchilada sauce

8 burrito-size whole-wheat tortillas

½ cup (58 g) shredded Monterey Jack cheese

① Spray a 9-inch (23 cm) baking dish with nonstick cooking spray.

② Chop mushrooms and set aside. Heat olive oil in a large nonstick skillet over medium-high heat. Add garlic and cook, stirring constantly, for 1 minute.

③ Add mushrooms, thyme, salt, and pepper and cook, stirring often, until mushrooms release their moisture and become tender and browned, about 7 minutes.

④ Transfer to a large mixing bowl and stir in cilantro, sour cream, and Neufchâtel, allowing the cheese to melt and the mixture to get creamy.

⑤ Heat enchilada sauce in a large skillet over low heat. Dip a tortilla in sauce to coat both sides and allow excess sauce to drip off.

⑥ Lay tortilla in the baking dish and fill with mushroom mixture, rolling tortilla around filling and placing enchilada seam-side down against the side of the baking dish. Repeat with remaining tortillas and mushroom mixture. Pour remaining enchilada sauce evenly over tortillas and sprinkle with Monterey Jack cheese. Let cool completely.

YIELD: 10 SERVINGS

## COOKING TIP: TRY WILD MUSHROOMS

Wild mushrooms can be sautéed, broiled, grilled, baked, roasted, and some, like enoki, can be deliciously eaten raw. Their meaty texture and savory flavors add unparalleled dimension to any dish they grace and best yet, for relatively few calories and carbs. In vegetarian dishes, wild mushrooms mimic the texture of beef and poultry, making them a star ingredient for new vegetarians or for meat-eating guests who come to dinner.

 ## TO FREEZE

Spray a piece of heavy-duty aluminum foil with nonstick cooking spray and tightly cover baking dish with cooking spray-side down (this will keep the cheese from sticking to the foil). Place in the freezer.

 ## TO REHEAT

Let enchiladas thaw in the refrigerator overnight.

OVEN METHOD: Preheat oven to 350°F (180°C, or gas mark 4) and bake for 30 minutes. Remove foil and bake for an additional 10 minutes or until cheese is bubbly and lightly browned.

AMOUNT PER SERVING: Calories 512.24; Total Fat 16.89 g; Cholesterol 31.77 mg; Sodium 812.50 mg; Potassium 1455.64 mg; Total Carbohydrates 85.07 g; Fiber 16.76 g; Sugar 3 g; Protein 16.19 g

# VEGGIE AND BLACK BEAN TORTILLA BAKE

This particular dish is a favorite because not only does it boast all of the classic Mexican flavors, it is chock-full of vegetables and beans—a healthy vegetarian meal when I feel the need to bolster my son's vegetable intake.

2 tablespoons (28 ml) olive oil

1 onion, diced

1 large red bell pepper, seeded, diced

6 cups (420 g) shredded cabbage

1 can (28 ounces, or 785 g) fire-roasted diced tomatoes, or 3¾ cups (675 g) Fire-Roasted Tomatoes (see below)

1½ cups (360 g) red enchilada sauce

1 tablespoon (7 g) Hot and Healthy Spice Blend (page 171)

3 cans (15 ounces, or 425 g, each) black beans, rinsed, drained

¼ cup (4 g) finely chopped cilantro

Salt and freshly ground black pepper

12 ounces (340 g) Neufchâtel cheese, softened at room temperature

½ cup (115 g) plain Greek yogurt

Grated zest and juice of 1 lime

2 cans (7 ounces, or 200 g, each) diced green chiles

10 whole-grain flour tortillas

1½ cups (173 g) shredded Monterey Jack cheese

① Preheat oven to 350°F (180°C, or gas mark 4) and grease a 13 x 9-inch (33 x 23 cm) baking dish.

② Heat oil in a large skillet over medium heat. Add onion, pepper, and cabbage and cook, stirring often, until vegetables are tender and lightly browned.

③ Add tomatoes, enchilada sauce, Hot and Healthy Spice Blend, stirring to combine. Bring to a boil and reduce heat to medium-low. Simmer for 5 minutes. Stir in beans and cilantro. Season with salt and pepper. Set aside.

④ In the bowl of a food processor, combine Neufchâtel, yogurt, and lime zest and juice, and process until smooth. Add chiles and pulse a few times just to combine.

⑤ Cut the tortillas in half and line the bottom of the baking dish with ten halves. Dollop cheese mixture over tortillas and top with a layer of bean sauce. Repeat with remaining tortillas, cheese, and black bean sauce. Sprinkle with shredded cheese. Spray one side of a sheet of foil and cover baking dish, spray-side down.

⑥ Bake for 30 minutes. Remove foil and bake 10 more minutes. Let cool completely.

YIELD: 8 SERVINGS

## COOKING TIP: FIRE-ROASTED TOMATOES

To fire roast tomatoes: Preheat your grill to medium heat. Slice Roma tomatoes in half lengthwise and rub with olive oil. Season lightly with salt and freshly ground black pepper. Place tomatoes in a grill basket and set over the heat. Grill, flipping occasionally, until the tomato skins are lightly blackened. Set them in a bowl and cover with plastic wrap; this will steam the tomatoes so the skins are easy to remove. Peel off most of the skins. Spread tomatoes and their juices on a baking sheet and allow to cool completely.

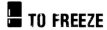 TO FREEZE

INDIVIDUAL SERVINGS: Divide casserole among 8 freezer- and microwave-safe containers.

FOR A CROWD: Cover dish with freezer wrap.

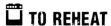 TO REHEAT

Let casserole thaw in the refrigerator overnight.

MICROWAVE METHOD: Reheat individual servings in the microwave on high for 2 minutes or until heated through.

OVEN METHOD: Preheat oven to 375°F (190°C, or gas mark 5). Remove freezer wrap from dish and cover with foil. Bake for 20 minutes. Uncover and bake 10 minutes more.

AMOUNT PER SERVING: Calories 796.02; Total Fat 28.84 g; Cholesterol 52.41 mg; Sodium 1422.42 mg; Potassium 2473.66 mg; Total Carbohydrates 108.2 g; Fiber 43.89 g; Sugar 34.04 g; Protein 34.35 g

# CHAPTER 3

# MEATS
## MOUTHWATERING MEAL CENTERPIECES TO PLEASE ANY PALATE

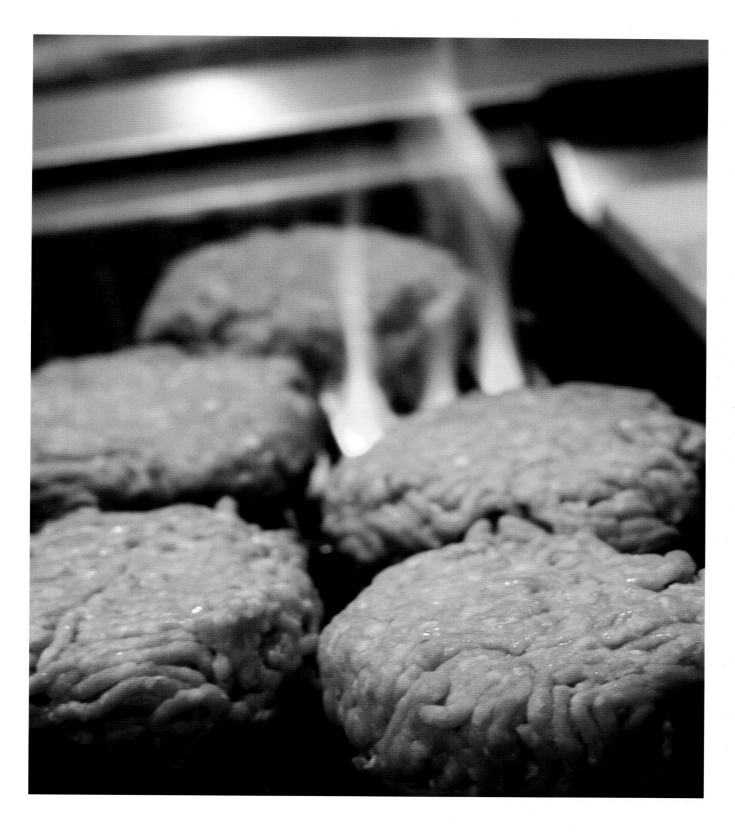

# SLIM AND TRIM BEEF AND PAPAYA BURRITOS

Adding fruit to savory meals lends a contrast of flavor while also helping your family meet the daily 5 to 9 servings of fruits and vegetables recommended for optimal health. These lean beef burritos are bursting with sweet, spicy, and tangy flavors. The creative combination of papaya, warm spices, and goat cheese will have your attention at first bite.

**2 tablespoons (28 ml) canola oil**

**2 pounds (910 g) extra-lean ground beef (96/4)**

**1 onion, chopped**

**3 cloves garlic, minced**

**Pinch of salt**

**Freshly ground black pepper to taste**

**2 tablespoons (18 g) chipotle peppers in adobo sauce, finely chopped**

**1 teaspoon ground cumin**

**1 teaspoon ground coriander**

**1½ cups (265 g) diced fresh papaya**

**¼ cup (4 g) finely chopped fresh cilantro**

**1 cup (150 g) crumbled goat cheese**

**8 to 10 whole-grain burrito-size flour tortillas**

① Heat oil in a Dutch oven over medium-high heat. Add beef and onion and cook, stirring often to break up beef, until beef is browned and onion is soft. Add garlic, salt, pepper, chipotle, cumin, and coriander and cook, stirring often, for 1 minute.

② Stir in papaya and cook, stirring occasionally, for 3 to 4 minutes or until fruit is softened. Stir in cilantro and goat cheese. Remove from heat and allow to cool completely.

③ For each burrito, place beef filling in the center of the tortilla and then fold the top and bottom edges over and roll burrito-style.

YIELD: 8 TO 10 BURRITOS, OR 8 SERVINGS

## COOKING TIP: GET CREATIVE WITH LEFTOVER PAPAYA

- Combine chunks of papaya, pineapple, and banana and toss with lime juice and shredded sweetened coconut.
- Add it to your green or grain salads.
- Purée it with agave to taste, adding enough water to thin slightly, and serve as a chilled soup.
- Bake it sprinkled with a little brown sugar and cinnamon and serve it as a warm side dish.
- Crush it with honey and simmer into a sauce to pour over ice cream and cake.

 **TO FREEZE**

INDIVIDUAL SERVINGS: Tightly wrap each burrito with freezer wrap.

FOR A CROWD: Place burritos in a baking dish or on a baking sheet, leaving room in between each burrito. Freeze until solid. Transfer burritos to 1-gallon (3.8 L) freezer bags, removing as much air as possible before sealing.

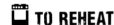 **TO REHEAT**

Let burritos thaw in refrigerator overnight.

MICROWAVE METHOD: Individual burritos can be heated in the microwave on high for 2 to 3 minutes or until heated through.

OVEN METHOD: Preheat oven to 350°F (180°C, or gas mark 4). Place burritos in a single layer in a baking dish. Cover dish with foil and bake for 15 to 20 minutes or until heated through.

AMOUNT PER SERVING: Calories 310.11; Total Fat 11.3 g; Cholesterol 63.32 mg; Sodium 161.4 mg; Potassium 537.4 mg; Total Carbohydrates 26.38 g; Fiber 4.51 g; Sugar 2.33 g; Protein 26.83 g

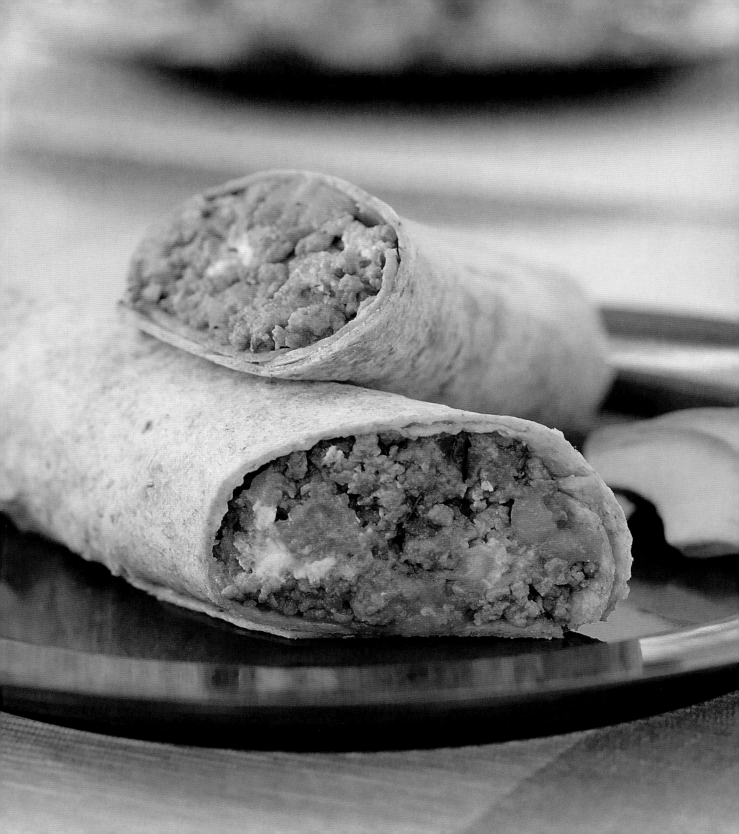

# FREEZER-FABULOUS GORGONZOLA BURGERS

Simple, succulent, and hands down the go-to meal when you want a healthy gourmet meal, these grilled gorgonzola burgers are especially delicious when topped off with a layer of antioxidant-rich roasted red peppers. Partner up with a whole-grain bun, and you've got the perfect lunch or dinner.

**2 pounds (900 g) extra-lean ground beef**

**½ teaspoon salt**

**Freshly ground black pepper to taste**

**2 teaspoons (4 g) Italian seasoning**

**8 ounces (225 g) gorgonzola cheese**

① Preheat grill to medium-high heat.

② In a large bowl, mix together beef, salt, pepper, and Italian seasoning. Shape into 16 same-size patties.

③ Place 1 ounce (28 g) crumbled gorgonzola on 8 of the patties, spreading it out almost to the edges. Place remaining patties on top, pressing down and sealing edges.

④ Oil the grate and grill burgers for 4 to 5 minutes per side or until desired doneness. Transfer to a wire rack and allow to cool completely.

YIELD: 8 BURGERS, OR 8 SERVINGS

## BONUS RECIPE

Top burgers with Roasted Red Pepper Sauce (below) and Best By the Batch Caramelized Onions (page 104).

Roasted Red Pepper Sauce

- 1 cup (180 g) Roasted Red Peppers (page 139)
- 1 clove garlic, crushed
- 2 tablespoons (8 g) fresh parsley
- 1 tablespoon (6 g) lemon zest
- Juice of half of a lemon
- Salt and freshly ground black pepper to taste
- ½ cup (115 g) Greek yogurt

Purée first 5 ingredients. Season with salt and pepper. Add yogurt and blend until well-combined.

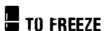 **TO FREEZE**

Place burgers on a baking sheet and freeze until firm. Wrap each burger in freezer wrap and place in a 1-gallon (3.8 L) freezer bag.

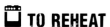 **TO REHEAT**

Let burgers thaw in refrigerator overnight.

MICROWAVE METHOD: Reheat burgers in the microwave on 60% power for 1 to 2 minutes or until heated through. Don't overcook.

OVEN METHOD: Preheat oven to 375°F (190°C, or gas mark 5). Place burgers on a baking sheet and cook for 10 minutes or until heated through.

AMOUNT PER SERVING: Calories 257.91; Total Fat 14.8 g; Cholesterol 95.86 mg; Sodium 615.64 mg; Potassium 393.61 mg; Total Carbohydrates 0.99 g; Fiber 0 g; Sugar 0 g; Protein 30.43 g

# BETTER-THAN-TAKEOUT ASIAN BEEF STRIPS

Lean beef marinated in Asian flavors and steamed brown basmati rice makes for a fabulous lunch or dinner far healthier than ordering takeout. If you have it on hand, swap in Ginger and Veggie Fried Rice (page 111) for the basmati rice. Serve with Naturally Sweet Agave-Glazed Carrots (page 101) or Fast-Fix Zucchini Slaw (page 102).

½ cup (120 ml) fresh-squeezed orange juice

1 tablespoon (6 g) minced orange zest

1 tablespoon (6 g) minced fresh peeled ginger

2 tablespoons (28 ml) rice wine vinegar

3 tablespoons (45 ml) shoyu

2 tablespoons (40 g) honey

Pinch of hot red pepper flakes

2 pounds (900 g) flank steak, sliced diagonally into ¼-inch (6 mm) slices

1 tablespoon (8 g) cornstarch

1 tablespoon (15 ml) canola oil

1 tablespoon (15 ml) sesame oil

4 cups (780 g) cooked brown basmati rice, cooled completely

① In a large bowl, whisk together orange juice, orange zest, ginger, vinegar, shoyu, honey, and red pepper flakes. Place steak in bowl and toss to coat. Cover bowl and refrigerate for 2 hours.

② Remove meat from the marinade and whisk cornstarch into the marinade. Heat oil in a wok over medium-high heat. Swirl to coat.

③ Stir-fry the meat for 2 to 3 minutes. Add marinade and cook, stirring, until sauce is thickened. Drizzle with sesame oil. Remove from heat and let cool completely.

YIELD: 8 SERVINGS

## COOKING TIP: FREEZE CITRUS ZEST

To ensure you always have vibrant citrus zest on hand, keep zest (and juice) in the freezer. To freeze zest: Use a citrus zester or grater and remove the colorful peel, avoiding the bitter white pith underneath. Lay zest on a sheet of waxed paper and freeze. Scrape frozen zest into a freezer bag, removing as much air as possible before sealing.

 ## TO FREEZE

INDIVIDUAL SERVINGS: Divide steak and rice into 1-quart (950 ml) freezer bags or freezer- and microwave-safe containers.

FOR A CROWD: Place steak and rice in 2 separate 1-gallon (3.8 L) freezer bags, removing as much air as possible before sealing.

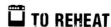 ## TO REHEAT

Let steak and rice thaw in refrigerator overnight.

MICROWAVE METHOD: Reheat individual servings in the microwave on high for 2 to 3 minutes or until heated through.

OVEN METHOD: Preheat oven to 350°F (180°C, or gas mark 4). Place rice in a baking dish and top with steak. Cover with foil and bake for 20 minutes or until heated through.

AMOUNT PER SERVING: Calories 332.61; Total Fat 13.6 g; Cholesterol 46.64 mg; Sodium 268.07 mg; Potassium 482.68 mg; Total Carbohydrates 26.22 g; Fiber 1.54 g; Sugar 5.81 g; Protein 26.54 g

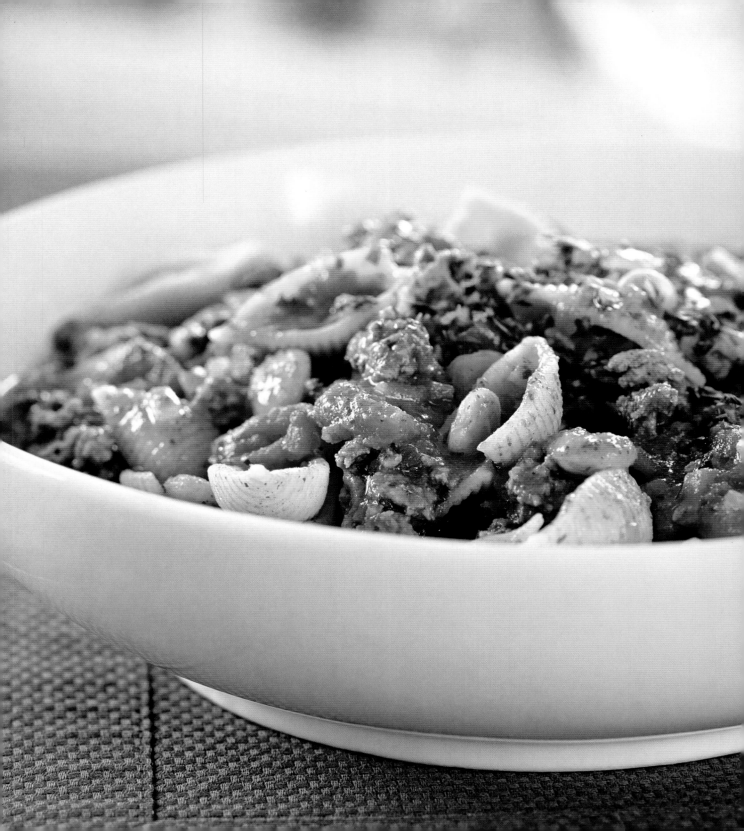

# HOT AND SPICY BORBOA GOULASH

When I was growing up, goulash was one of those intoxicatingly fragrant meals that led my family to the dinner table by the nose and then warmed every bone in our bodies with the richly spiced meat, tomatoes, and tender pasta shells. Over the years, I've made a few modifications to make it healthier, and it remains one of my favorite comfort foods.

2 tablespoons (28 ml) olive oil

2 pounds (900 g) extra-lean ground beef

1 green bell pepper, seeded, diced

1 onion, diced

2 jalapeños, seeded, minced

Salt and freshly ground black pepper

2 tablespoons (16 g) chili powder (or to taste)

1 teaspoon ground cinnamon

1 teaspoon ground cumin

1 teaspoon ground coriander

3 cans (15 ounces, or 425 g, each) stewed tomatoes (do not drain)

1 pound (455 g) whole-wheat pasta shells

2 cups (340 g) lima beans

¼ cup (4 g) finely chopped fresh cilantro

① Heat oil in a stockpot over medium heat. Add beef, green pepper, onion, and jalapeño and cook, stirring often, until beef is browned and vegetables are tender. Season with salt and pepper, chili powder, cinnamon, cumin, and coriander, stirring to combine. Add stewed tomatoes and bring to a low boil. Reduce heat to medium-low and simmer for 15 minutes, stirring occasionally.

② Cook pasta in salted boiling water for 1 to 2 minutes less than package directions. Drain and add to beef mixture. Stir in lima beans. If mixture seems too thick, stir in ½ cup (120 ml) or so of water and simmer for 5 more minutes. Stir in cilantro and remove from heat. Let cool completely.

YIELD: 8 SERVINGS

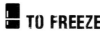 TO FREEZE

INDIVIDUAL SERVINGS: Divide goulash into 8 freezer- and microwave-safe containers.

FOR A CROWD: Transfer goulash to a large freezer bag, seal, and lay flat in a baking dish. Freeze until solid, and then remove baking dish.

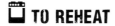 TO REHEAT

Let goulash thaw in the refrigerator overnight.

MICROWAVE METHOD: Reheat individual servings of goulash in the microwave on high, stirring every minute, for 2 minutes or until heated through.

STOVETOP METHOD: Reheat goulash in a stockpot over medium-high heat, stirring occasionally, for 10 minutes or until heated through.

AMOUNT PER SERVING: Calories 471.1; Total Fat 10.74 g; Cholesterol 70.53 mg; Sodium 560.79 mg; Potassium 901.18 mg; Total Carbohydrates 60.9 g; Fiber 6.82 g; Sugar 8.43g; Protein 35 g

# MAKE-IT-A-MEAL MEATLOAF

Made with a medley of lower-fat ground meat and finely chopped fruit and vegetables makes this meatloaf a healthy alternative to the usual fat-dripping, bacon-covered varieties. For a change, substitute beef or pork with ground turkey.

1 pound (455 g) extra-lean ground beef

1 pound (455 g) ground pork

2 eggs

2 tablespoons (22 g) Dijon mustard

½ cup (60 g) dry whole-wheat bread crumbs

3 scallions, minced (green and white parts)

2 carrots, minced

1 cup dried cherries, minced

1 tablespoon (6 g) Italian seasoning

Pinch of cayenne

Salt and freshly ground black pepper to taste

① Preheat oven to 350°F (180°C, or gas mark 4) and grease a large loaf pan.

② In a large bowl, combine all ingredients. Transfer to prepared loaf pan, firmly packing. Bake for 75 minutes. Set on a wire rack to cool for 15 minutes. Invert onto a wire rack and cool completely. (If you are freezing as individual servings, cut meatloaf into 8 slices to cool quicker.)

YIELD: 1 LOAF, OR 8 SERVINGS

**SERVING SUGGESTIONS TO MAKE YOUR MEATLOAF A BALANCED MEAL:**

- Nestle it between slices of Whole-Grain Seeded Bread (page 128) and a green salad.
- Serve it with Smashed Garlic Potatoes (page 108) and Naturally Sweet Agave-Glazed Carrots (page 101).
- Try it with Tender Roasted Vegetables (page 105) and Soft and Seeded Oat Knots (page 142).
- Pair it with Apricot-Pistachio Rice Pilaf (page 113) and Fast and Fabulous Fava Beans (page 106).
- Serve it with a side of pasta tossed with Five-Ways Fresh Herb Spread (page 170) and Best by the Batch Caramelized Onions (page 104).

 **TO FREEZE**

INDIVIDUAL SERVINGS: Wrap individual slices with freezer wrap.

FOR A CROWD: Wrap meatloaf with freezer wrap.

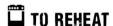 **TO REHEAT**

Let meatloaf thaw in refrigerator overnight. For whole meatloaf, remove freezer wrap and set meatloaf in original loaf pan before thawing.

MICROWAVE METHOD: Microwave individual slices on high for 2 minutes or until heated through.

OVEN METHOD: Preheat oven to 375°F (190°C, or gas mark 5). Bake meatloaf for 30 minutes or until heated through.

AMOUNT PER SERVING: Calories 345.66; Total Fat 16.99 g; Cholesterol 129.09 mg; Sodium 200.73 mg; Potassium 476.03 mg; Total Carbohydrates 22.7 g; Fiber 2.17 g; Sugar 1.61 g; Protein 25.24 g

# SLOW COOKER SHREDDED BEEF

Shredded beef is an ultra-versatile staple to have in your freezer to quickly feed a crowd. This recipe calls for onion soup mix, but you can season the beef in a variety of ways depending on how you plan to serve it.

**1 brisket (3½ pounds, or 1.6 kg), untrimmed**

**1 package (1 ounce, or 28 g) onion soup mix**

**Grated zest and juice from 1 large lemon**

**1 tablespoon (8 g) cornstarch**

**2 tablespoons (28 ml) water**

① Place brisket in a slow cooker and rub with soup mix, lemon zest, and juice. Turn brisket fat-side up and cook on low for 8 to 10 hours. (Hint: Cook it overnight so it's ready to be cooled in the morning.)

② Remove brisket from slow cooker and peel off fat. Set aside until cool enough to handle. Shred beef. Pour juices from slow cooker into a baking dish and let cool completely.

YIELD: 16 SERVINGS

## SERVING SUGGESTIONS

- Toss shredded beef with barbecue sauce and pile it on Honey Whole-Wheat Freezer Rolls (page 129) and Fast-Fix Zucchini Slaw (page 102).
- Tuck it in tortillas with shredded cabbage, sour cream, and fruit salsa.
- Use it in place of ground beef in enchiladas.
- Make enchiladas by mixing shredded beef with Best by the Batch Caramelized Onions (page 104), Fire-Roasted Tomatoes (page 39), scallions, and feta. Roll into tortillas, top with enchilada sauce and cheese and bake.

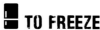 **TO FREEZE**

INDIVIDUAL SERVINGS: Divide beef into 16 freezer- and microwave-safe containers or 1-quart (950 ml) freezer bags. Add 2 tablespoons (28 ml) of juices to each and seal.

FOR A CROWD: Place beef in a 1-gallon (3.8 L) freezer bag and remove as much as air as possible before sealing and laying flat in the freezer. Place juices in a freezer bag, removing as much air as possible before sealing, and lay flat in a baking dish. Freeze until solid and then remove baking dish.

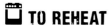 **TO REHEAT**

Let beef and juices thaw in the refrigerator overnight.

MICROWAVE METHOD: Individual servings of beef can be reheated in the microwave on high for 2 minutes or until heated through.

STOVETOP METHOD: Place beef in a large skillet over medium heat and cook, stirring, until heated through. Place juices in a saucepan over medium-high heat. Whisk together 1 tablespoon (8 g) cornstarch and 2 tablespoons (28 ml) water. Whisk cornstarch into juices and bring to a boil. Cook, stirring, until thickened. Use as gravy.

AMOUNT PER SERVING: Calories 206.38; Total Fat 14.92 g; Cholesterol 54 mg; Sodium 1357.79 mg; Potassium 319.42 mg; Total Carbohydrates 2.45 g; Fiber 0.43 g; Sugar 0.08 g; Protein 14.89 g

# HEALTHY MEAT AND (SWEET) POTATOES

Meat and potatoes is an American staple that usually features high-fat beef and fried potatoes. These scrumptious meat-stuffed sweet potatoes have fewer calories and fat grams while providing far more fiber and disease-fighting antioxidants.

**8 small sweet potatoes**

**2 tablespoons (28 ml) olive oil, divided**

**Salt and freshly ground black pepper to taste**

**1 pound (455 g) extra-lean ground beef or ground pork**

**1 onion, chopped**

**2 cloves garlic, minced**

**1 can (15 ounces, or 455 g) kidney beans, rinsed, drained**

**1 can (16 ounces, or 454 g) tomato sauce**

**1 cup (275 g) chili sauce**

**1 tablespoon (6 g) Italian seasoning**

① Preheat oven to 400°F (200°C, or gas mark 6). Rub sweet potatoes with 1 tablespoon (15 ml) olive oil. Rub with salt and pepper. Place potatoes on a baking sheet and bake for 50 minutes or until potatoes give when pressed. Remove from the oven and let cool completely on a wire rack.

② Heat 1 tablespoon (15 ml) oil in a large skillet over medium-high heat. Add beef or pork and onion and cook, stirring often, until beef is browned and onion is soft. Add garlic and cook, stirring often, for 1 minute. Season with salt and pepper.

③ Add beans, tomato sauce, chili sauce, and Italian seasoning, stirring to combine. Bring to a boil, stirring occasionally, and then lower heat and simmer for 5 minutes. Remove from heat and let cool completely.

YIELD: 8 SERVINGS

 ## TO FREEZE

INDIVIDUAL SERVINGS: Wrap each potato in freezer wrap. Divide beef mixture among 8 freezer- and microwave-safe containers or 1-quart (950 ml) freezer bags, removing as much air as possible before sealing.

FOR A CROWD: Place potatoes on a baking sheet and freeze until firm. Transfer to large freezer bags, removing as much air as possible before sealing. Transfer beef mixture to a large freezer bag, removing as much air as possible before sealing, and then lay in a baking dish. Freeze until solid and then remove baking dish.

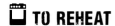 ## TO REHEAT

Let potatoes and meat mixture thaw in refrigerator overnight.

MICROWAVE METHOD: Split open a potato and top with meat mixture. Microwave on 70% power for 3 to 4 minutes or until heated through.

OVEN METHOD: Preheat oven to 375°F (190°C, or gas mark 5). Place potatoes in a baking dish and cover with foil. Place meat mixture in a baking dish and cover with foil. Bake for 25 minutes or until heated through. To serve, split potatoes open and fill with meat mixture. Top with shredded cheese if desired.

AMOUNT PER SERVING: Calories 320.33; Total Fat 6.55 g; Cholesterol 35.26 mg; Sodium 989.98 mg; Potassium 1111.18 mg; Total Carbohydrates 46.2 g; Fiber 10 g; Sugar 13.11 g; Protein 18.87 g

# ASIAN PORK AND 5-SPICE APPLES

Pork and apple gets an Asian twist with Chinese 5-Spice powder, sesame oil, and black vinegar. Low in fat, strips of pork loin are a palate-pleasing source of lean protein that pairs impeccably with tender, unusually spiced apples.

2 tablespoons (28 ml) black vinegar or balsamic vinegar

2 tablespoons (28 ml) dry sherry

1 tablespoon (15 ml) sesame oil

1 tablespoon (15 ml) tamari

1 tablespoon (5 g) cracked black peppercorns

3 tablespoons (12 g) chopped fresh tarragon leaves

2 cloves garlic, minced

2 pounds (900 g) boneless pork loin, cut into strips

2 tablespoons (28 ml) canola oil

3 Golden Delicious apples, cored, halved, sliced

1 teaspoon Chinese 5-Spice powder

2 tablespoons (30 g) packed brown sugar

¼ cup (60 ml) freshly squeezed orange juice

1 tablespoon (8 g) cornstarch

3 tablespoons (9 g) minced chives

4 cups (780 g) cooked brown rice, cooled

① In a large bowl, whisk together vinegar, sherry, sesame oil, tamari, peppercorns, tarragon, and garlic. Reserve ½ cup (120 ml) marinade and refrigerate. Add pork and toss to coat. Cover and refrigerate for 2 to 3 hours.

② Heat oil in a wok over medium-high heat, add apples, and stir-fry for 2 minutes. Sprinkle with 5-Spice, brown sugar, and orange juice and continue to stir-fry for 2 to 3 minutes.

③ Remove pork from marinade, allowing the excess to drip off. Add pork to the wok and cook, stirring often, for 2 to 3 minutes or until pork is just cooked through.

④ Whisk cornstarch into reserved marinade and stir into pork mixture until thickened. Remove from heat and stir in chives. Cool completely.

YIELD: 8 SERVINGS

## COOKING TIP: EXPERIMENT WITH 5-SPICE POWDER

Available in Chinese markets and the spice aisle or Asian section of most major supermarkets, 5-Spice powder is a distinctively flavored blend of 5 spices: star anise, cloves, cinnamon, fennel, and Sichuan pepper. Used mostly in savory Asian dishes, it adds an unusual yet welcome flavor to desserts. Stir it into softened vanilla ice cream or use a dash to add a surprising taste to fruit salads.

 ## TO FREEZE

INDIVIDUAL SERVINGS: Divide pork mixture and rice into freezer- and microwave-safe containers.

FOR A CROWD: Place pork mixture and rice into 2 separate 1-gallon (3.8 L) freezer bags.

 ## TO REHEAT

Let pork and rice thaw in the refrigerator overnight.

MICROWAVE METHOD: Reheat individual portions in the microwave on high for 2 to 3 minutes or until heated through.

OVEN METHOD: Preheat oven to 350°F (180°C, or gas mark 4). Place rice in a baking dish and cover with pork mixture. Cover with foil and bake for 20 to 25 minutes or until heated through.

AMOUNT PER SERVING:  Calories 338.98; Total Fat 9.95 g; Cholesterol 75.08 mg; Sodium 191.18 mg; Potassium 586.75 mg; Total Carbohydrates 32.24 g; Fiber 3.34 g; Sugar 8.68 g; Protein 28.59 g

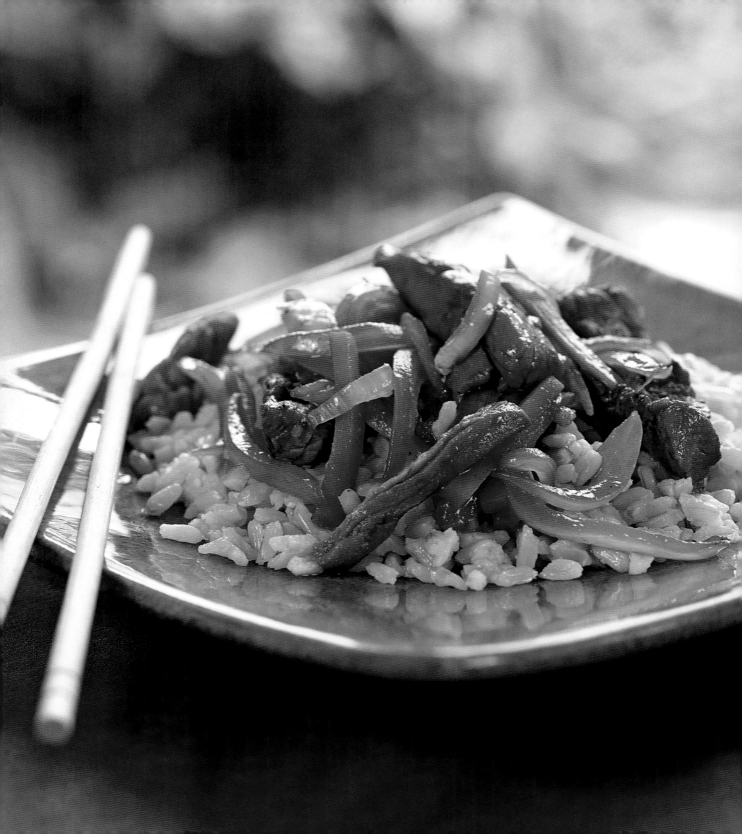

# GOOD-FOR-YOU MU SHU PORK

When the craving hits for Chinese food, pull this Mu Shu Pork out of the freezer. Tender strips of pork and shredded vegetables in an Asian sauce far surpasses supermarket freezer main courses or takeout when it comes to a healthy meal.

**2 pounds (900 g) pork tenderloin, cut into strips**

**½ cup (120 ml) tamari**

**2 tablespoons (28 ml) sesame oil**

**3 cloves garlic, crushed**

**Juice and grated zest of 2 limes**

**2 tablespoons (16 g) All-Purpose Asian Spice Blend (page 174)**

**2 tablespoons (28 ml) canola oil**

**1 onion, halved, thinly sliced**

**1 small head napa cabbage, shredded or very thinly sliced crosswise**

**3 carrots, shredded or cut into matchsticks**

**½ cup (125 ml) hoisin sauce**

**8 cups (1.3 kg) Ginger and Veggie Fried Rice (page 111) or Family Favorite Freezer Rice (page 110)**

① Place pork in a 1-gallon (3.8 L) bag. In a small bowl, whisk together tamari, sesame oil, garlic, lime juice and zest, and Asian Spice Blend. Pour into bag, seal, and rub marinade into pork. Refrigerate for at least 2 hours or overnight.

② Heat canola oil in a wok or large nonstick skillet over medium-high heat. Add pork and cook, stirring often, until browned and cooked through. Transfer to a plate. Add more oil to the wok or skillet, if needed.

③ Add onion, cabbage, and carrots to wok or skillet and cook, stirring often, until vegetables are tender. Add pork to vegetable mixture and stir in hoisin, tossing to coat pork and vegetables. Remove from heat and let cool completely.

YIELD: 8 SERVINGS

## COOKING TIP: KNOW YOUR SESAME OIL

Cold-pressed sesame oil: Light in color and mild in flavor, cold-pressed sesame oil has a high smoke point and can be used in high-heat cooking. Toasted sesame oil: Darker in color and richer in flavor, toasted sesame oil is best used for lower-heat cooking methods or added after cooking for flavor. Drizzle it over cooked foods or use it as a dipping sauce.

 ## TO FREEZE

INDIVIDUAL SERVINGS: If you are steaming rice while the pork is cooking, let rice cool completely. Place 1 cup (165 g) rice in each of 8 freezer- and microwave-safe containers. Divide pork mixture among containers and freeze.

FOR A CROWD: If you are steaming rice while pork is cooking, let rice cool completely. Place rice in a 1-gallon (3.8 L) freezer bag, removing as much air as possible before sealing. Place pork mixture in a second 1-gallon (3.8 L) freezer bag, removing as much as possible before sealing.

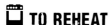 ## TO REHEAT

Let pork and rice thaw in the refrigerator overnight.

MICROWAVE METHOD: Place individual servings of pork and rice mixture in the microwave and reheat on high, stirring every minute, for 2 to 3 minutes or until heated through.

OVEN METHOD: Preheat oven to 350°F (180°C, or gas mark 4). Place rice in the bottom of a baking dish. Pour pork mixture overtop. Cover baking dish with foil and bake for 20 to 25 minutes or until heated through.

AMOUNT PER SERVING: Calories 360.35; Total Fat 16.38 g; Cholesterol 107.41 mg; Sodium 1379.3 mg; Potassium 722.96 mg; Total Carbohydrates 15.29 g; Fiber 2.48 g; Sugar 7.47 g; Protein 37.2 g

# PARTY-PERFECT PORK AND VEGGIE DUMPLINGS

Little purses of pork and shredded veggies, these dumplings are the perfect light meal. These dumplings also double as fun finger food as a first course or cocktail party appetizer.

8 ounces (227 g) reduced-fat ground pork sausage

1 tablespoon (6 g) minced fresh ginger

2 carrots, shredded

6 red radishes, grated

1 cup (70 g) shredded cabbage

3 scallions, minced (white and green parts)

Generous pinch of salt

2 teaspoons (28 ml) tamari

2 tablespoons (26 g) granulated sugar

2 tablespoons (2 g) finely chopped fresh cilantro

2 tablespoons (16 g) cornstarch

3 tablespoons (45 ml) water

1 teaspoon (15 ml) toasted sesame oil

1 package (12 ounces, or 340 g) wonton wrappers

1 egg, beaten

① Set up a bamboo steamer over boiling water.

② In a large skillet over medium-high heat, cook sausage, ginger, carrots, radishes, cabbage, scallions, and salt, stirring often, until sausage is browned and vegetables are softened. Add tamari, sugar, and cilantro, stirring to combine.

③ In a small bowl, whisk together cornstarch and water. Pour into pork mixture, stirring until thickened. Remove from heat and stir in sesame oil. Allow mixture to cool.

④ Lay wonton wrappers out on a flat surface. Place a spoonful of pork filling in the center of each wonton wrapper. Use your fingers to moisten edges with egg. Fold up sides of wontons to make dumplings, lightly squeezing the middle of the dumpling while tapping the bottom on a flat surface so the dumpling will stand upright.

⑤ Steam dumplings in bamboo steamer for 15 minutes. Set on paper towel-lined wire racks to cool completely.

YIELD: 48 DUMPLINGS, OR 8 SERVINGS

## SERVING SUGGESTIONS

Pork dumplings are especially delish dunked in a flavorful dipping sauce. Try store-bought chili sauce or oyster sauce or make your own such as Super-Fast Everyday Peanut Sauce (page 164). For a lighter sauce, whisk together tamari and a generous sprinkle of All-Purpose Asian Spice Blend (page 174). You can also serve dumplings as a soup by simmering them in vegetable broth.

## TO FREEZE

INDIVIDUAL SERVINGS: Arrange dumplings on a baking sheet and freeze until solid. Place six dumplings in each of eight 1-quart (946 ml) freezer bags or freezer- and microwave-safe containers.

FOR A CROWD: Transfer to freezer bags arranging in a single layer or a large freezer container, layering with waxed paper.

## TO REHEAT

If using the microwave method, let dumplings thaw in refrigerator overnight. If using bamboo steamer method, keep dumplings frozen until ready to cook.

MICROWAVE METHOD: In a microwave-safe container, place dumplings in a single layer. Add 2 to 3 tablespoons (28 to 45 ml) of water. Cover with a vented lid or cover with plastic wrap slashed a few times to vent. Microwave on high for 2 to 3 minutes or until dumplings are heated though.

BAMBOO STEAMER METHOD: Place a bamboo steamer over boiling water. Arrange dumplings in steamer in one layer and steam for 25 minutes or until heated through.

AMOUNT PER SERVING: Calories 252.83; Total Fat 7.84 g; Cholesterol 48.71 mg; Sodium 853.65 mg; Potassium 226.15 mg; Total Carbohydrates 33.95 g; Fiber 1.88 g; Sugar 4.88 g; Protein 11.15 g

# ZESTY MARINATED LAMB CHOPS

Grilled lamb chops are a special meal that isn't that difficult to prepare. Great for spring holidays, summer cookouts, and elegant fall or winter (weather permitting) dinners, keeping these in your freezer gives you a great grilled meal in minutes. Unlike other grilled foods in this book, lamb is best if grilled fresh instead of grilled first, and then placed in the freezer.

½ cup (120 ml) olive oil

¼ cup (60 ml) aged balsamic vinegar

Grated zest and juice of 1 orange

2 cloves garlic, minced

2 tablespoons (4 g) finely chopped fresh rosemary

Salt and freshly ground black pepper to taste

8 loin lamb chops, 1 to 1½ inches (2.5 to 3.8 cm) thick

① In a large shallow baking dish, whisk together oil, vinegar, orange zest and juice, garlic, rosemary, salt, and pepper. Add lamb chops, turning to coat, and refrigerate overnight.

YIELD: 8 LAMB CHOPS, OR 8 SERVINGS

## NUTRITION SPOTLIGHT: GRASSFED MEATS

Due to food safety issues as well as concern for the environment, more families are turning to meats, eggs, and dairy products from grassfed and pastured animals. Enriching your diet with grassfed and pastured animals is not only healthier, humane, and more environmentally friendly, it is also more delicious than eating animals confined to a feedlot or cages. Organic, pastured meats and other products may be more pricey than their conventionally raised counterparts, but the health benefits are worth it.

 **TO FREEZE**

INDIVIDUAL SERVINGS: Place chops in individual serving-size freezer-safe containers. Evenly pour marinade over each. Seal and freeze.

FOR A CROWD: Transfer marinade and chops to a large freezer-safe container and freeze.

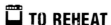 **TO REHEAT**

Let chops thaw in the refrigerator overnight. Allow them to come to room temperature before grilling to ensure even cooking.

GRILL METHOD: Preheat grill to medium-high heat. Oil grill grate and grill chops 7 to 8 minutes per side. Let rest for 5 minutes before serving.

AMOUNT PER SERVING: Calories 362.78; Total Fat 31.76 g; Cholesterol 56.88 mg; Sodium 49.38 mg; Potassium 232.53 mg; Total Carbohydrates 4.79 g; Fiber 0.97 g; Sugar 1.22 g; Protein 13.93 g

# BHUTANESE RED RICE AND LAMB

A relative newcomer to the United States, Bhutanese red rice is a red japonica rice that cooks into a pale pink, soft, and slightly sticky grain. This special rice is a nutty-flavored source of antioxidants, potassium, magnesium, and trace minerals and is a safe grain for gluten-free diets. You can find Bhutanese red rice in the grain section of Whole Foods stores and you can order online. If red rice is unavailable, simply use whatever rice you have on hand.

**1 bag (15 ounces, or 425 g) Bhutanese red rice**

**2 tablespoons (28 ml) olive oil**

**2 pounds (900 g) boneless lamb loin chops, chopped**

**Salt and freshly ground black pepper**

**1 onion, finely chopped**

**1 cup (100 g) chopped celery**

**1 cup (130 g) finely chopped carrots**

**2 zucchini, ends trimmed, diced**

**1 tablespoon (6 g) grated lemon zest**

**1 can (28 ounces, or 785 g) fire-roasted diced tomatoes, drained, or 3³⁄₄ cups (675 g) Fire-Roasted Tomatoes (page 39)**

**1 teaspoon sweet paprika**

**1 teaspoon Worcestershire sauce**

**1 tablespoon (2 g) fresh thyme leaves**

**2 tablespoons (8 g) finely chopped fresh parsley**

**³⁄₄ cup (113 g) crumbled feta cheese**

① Cook rice according to package directions. Set aside.

② Meanwhile, heat oil in a large pot over medium heat. Add lamb and cook, stirring often, until browned. Season with salt and pepper. Transfer to a plate.

③ Add onion, celery, carrot, and zucchini to pot and cook, stirring often, until softened and lightly browned. Season with salt and pepper.

④ Add rice, lamb, lemon zest, tomatoes, paprika, and Worcestershire sauce to pot, stirring to combine. Cook, stirring occasionally, for 2 to 3 minutes. Stir in thyme and parsley. Remove from heat and cool completely. Stir in feta.

YIELD: 10 SERVINGS

 ## TO FREEZE

INDIVIDUAL SERVINGS: Divide rice mixture into 10 freezer- and microwave-safe containers or 1-quart (950 ml) freezer bags, removing as much air as possible before sealing.

FOR A CROWD: Transfer rice mixture to a large freezer bag and lay in a casserole dish. Freeze until solid and then remove dish.

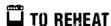 ## TO REHEAT

Let rice mixture thaw in refrigerator overnight.

MICROWAVE METHOD: Reheat individual servings of rice mixture in microwave on high, stirring every minute, for 2 to 3 minutes or until heated through.

OVEN METHOD: Preheat oven to 350°F (180°C, or gas mark 4). Place rice mixture in a baking dish, cover with foil, and bake for 30 minutes or until heated through.

AMOUNT PER SERVING: Calories 515.63; Total Fat 25.84 g; Cholesterol 75.57 mg; Sodium 207 mg; Potassium 830.8 mg; Total Carbohydrates 60.52 g; Fiber 8.04 g; Sugar 9.13 g; Protein 27.2 g

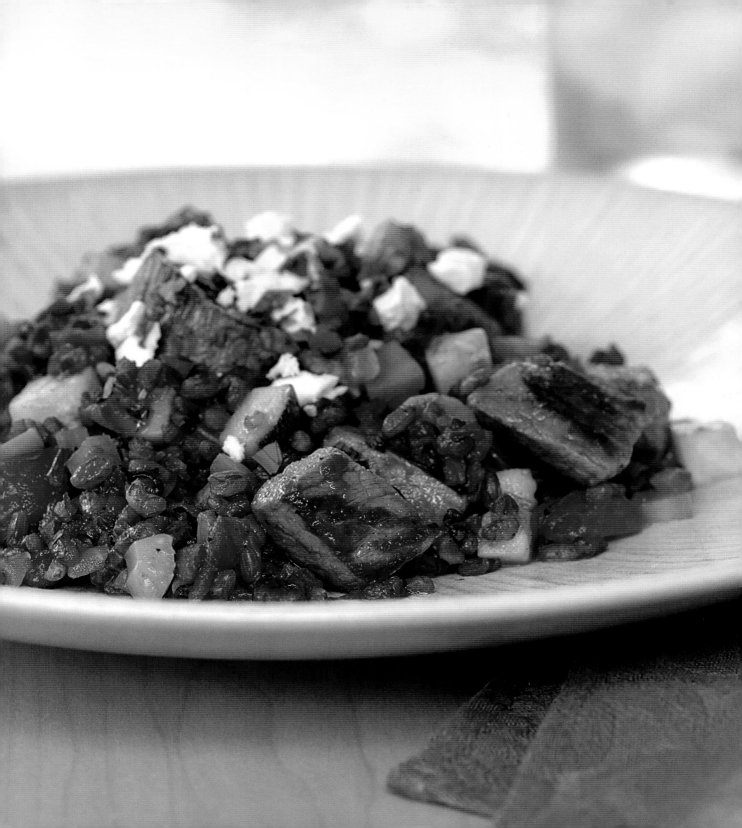

# CHAPTER 4

# POULTRY AND SEAFOOD
## LEAN-AND-MEAN MAIN DISHES

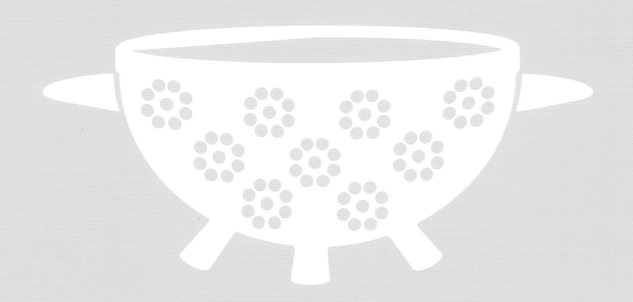

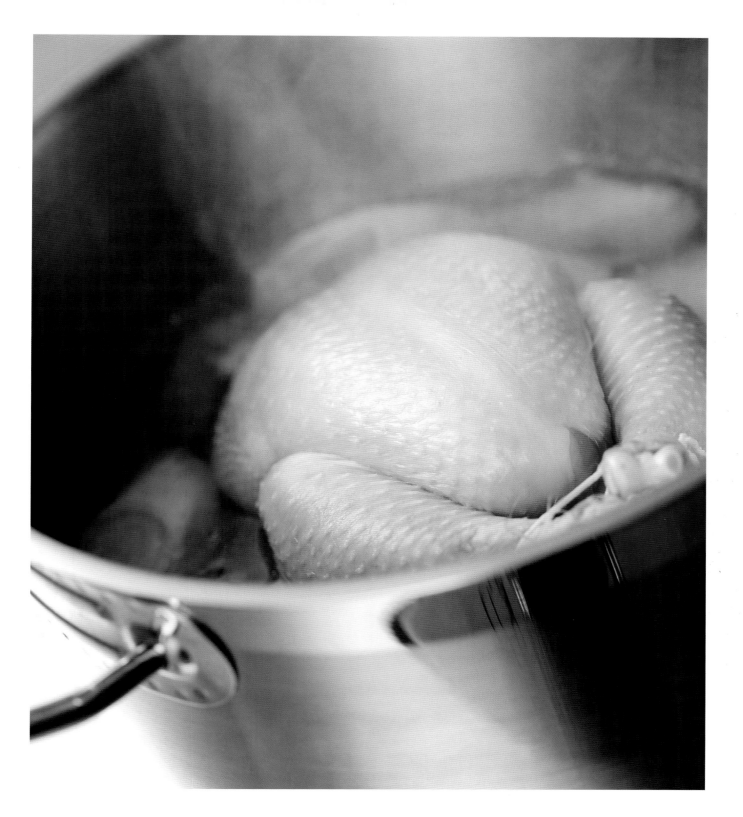

# COCONUT-CRUSTED CHICKEN STRIPS

It's time to break the drive-thru chicken nugget habit and serve your kids these crunchy baked chicken strips. Exceedingly lower in unhealthy fats and high in flavor, partner them with a low-fat ranch or honey mustard dressing.

**2 pounds (900 g) boneless, skinless chicken breasts**

**2 cups (230 g) blanched almond flour**

**1½ cups (120 g) shredded coconut**

**1 teaspoon salt**

**Freshly ground black pepper to taste**

**¼ teaspoon cayenne**

**1 teaspoon dried oregano**

**3 eggs**

① Preheat oven to 350°F (180°C, or gas mark 4) and spray 2 rimmed baking sheets with olive oil cooking spray.

② With the smooth side of a mallet or the bottom of a wide skillet, lightly pound chicken breasts to an even ½-inch (1.3 cm) thickness. Cut them into 1-inch (2.5 cm) wide strips. Set aside.

③ In a wide shallow dish, whisk together flour, coconut, salt, pepper, cayenne, and oregano. In a second shallow dish, beat eggs.

④ Dip chicken strips in egg mixture, allowing excess to drip off, and then coat on all sides in coconut mixture. Set on baking sheet. Spray chicken strips with olive oil cooking spray. Bake for 25 minutes, rotating pans after 12 to 13 minutes, or until coating is toasted and chicken is cooked through. Let cool completely.

YIELD: 8 SERVINGS

 **TO FREEZE**

Place chicken strips on a baking sheet and freeze until solid. Transfer chicken strips to 1-gallon (3.8 L) freezer bags, removing as much air as possible before sealing.

 **TO REHEAT**

Let chicken strips thaw in refrigerator overnight.

MICROWAVE METHOD: For small servings (3 or 4 strips), reheat on high for 1 to 2 minutes or until heated through. Increase cooking time for larger servings.

OVEN METHOD: Preheat oven to 350°F (180°C, or gas mark 4). Place chicken strips on a baking sheet and bake for 10 to 15 minutes or until heated through.

## NUTRITION SPOTLIGHT: ALMOND FLOUR

High in antioxidants, protein, fiber, and heart-healthy fats, almond flour is a delicious option for gluten-free and lower-carb diets. It doesn't need to be combined with other flours for successful baking, and it can be transformed into breakfasts, savory main courses, desserts, and more.

AMOUNT PER SERVING: Calories 282.96; Total Fat 12.53 g; Cholesterol 94.44 mg; Sodium 416.02 mg; Potassium 195.79 mg; Total Carbohydrates 10.39 g; Fiber 2.97 g; Sugar 5.76 g; Protein 31.25 g

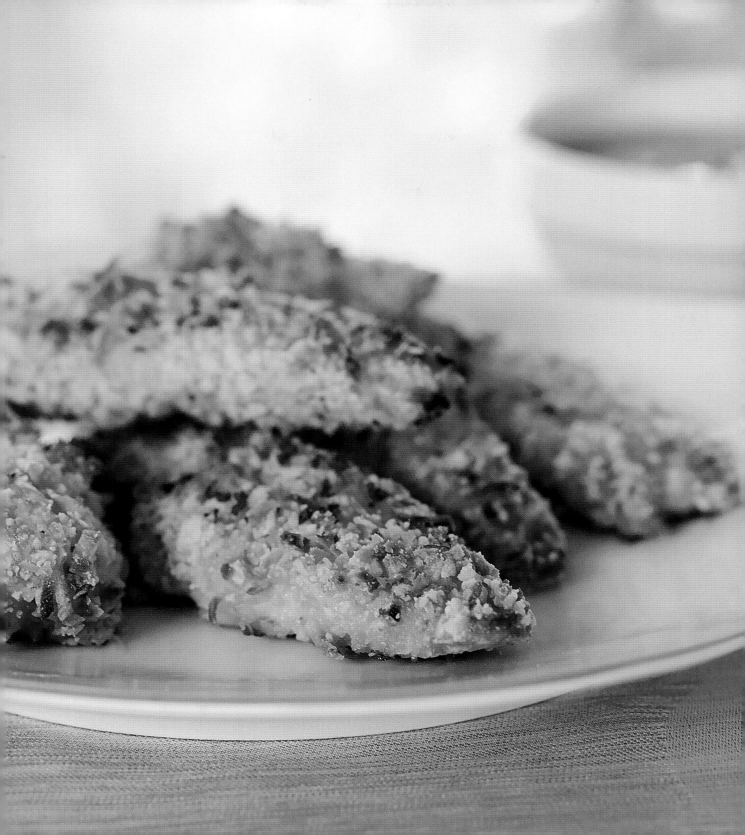

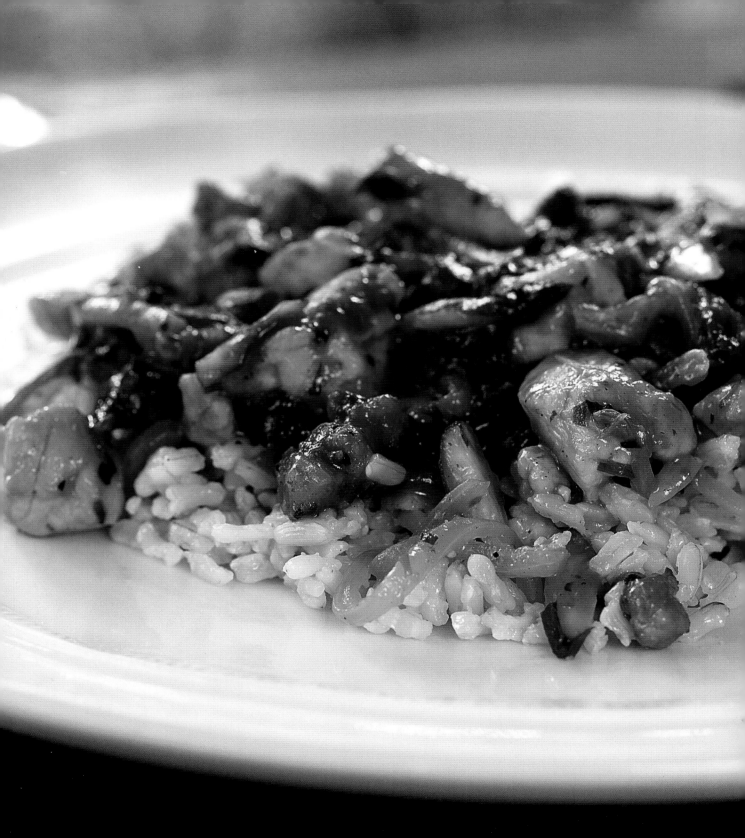

# SAUCY SAFFRON CHICKEN

Who says healthy weeknight dinners can't be special? Heady in fragrance and taste, saffron can make any meal gourmet. This fabulous chicken dish features an extra-flavorful combination of saffron, low-fat sausage, skinless chicken breast, almonds, and dried plums. Serve with Family-Favorite Freezer Rice (page 110) using your favorite long-grain rice.

**Pinch of saffron threads**

**¼ cup (60 ml) boiling water**

**1 cup (92 g) sliced almonds**

**2 tablespoons (28 ml) olive oil**

**4 ounces (115 g) low-fat turkey or chicken sausage, casing removed, sliced**

**1 large onion, quartered, thinly sliced**

**1½ pounds (680 g) boneless, skinless chicken breast, cubed**

**Salt and freshly ground black pepper to taste**

**Grated zest and juice of 1 lemon**

**1 cup (175 g) chopped dried plums**

**¼ cup (15 g) coarsely chopped fresh parsley**

**⅓ cup (80 ml) cold water**

**2 tablespoons (16 g) cornstarch** ›

**Family-Favorite Freezer Rice (page 110)**

① Crumble saffron in a small bowl with boiling water and set aside.

② Place a Dutch oven over medium heat. Add almonds and cook, stirring often, for 3 minutes or until just lightly toasted. Remove almonds and set aside.

③ Heat oil in Dutch oven and add sausage. Cook, stirring often, until browned. Remove with a slotted spoon and set aside. Add onion and cook, stirring often, until softened. Add chicken and cook, stirring occasionally, for 3 minutes. Season with salt and pepper.

④ Deglaze pan with saffron water, stirring to remove any browned bits on the bottom of the pan. Stir in lemon zest and juice, dried plums, and parsley.

⑤ Whisk together water and cornstarch. Pour into chicken mixture and bring to a boil. Cook, stirring occasionally, until thickened.

YIELD: 8 SERVINGS

 **TO FREEZE**

INDIVIDUAL SERVINGS: Allow mixture to cool completely. Divide chicken among 8 single-serving freezer and microwave-safe containers.

FOR A CROWD: Transfer chicken to a 1-gallon (3.8 L) freezer bag.

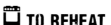 **TO REHEAT**

Take out desired amount (portions or entire recipe) and place in the refrigerator to defrost overnight.

MICROWAVE METHOD: Microwave for 2 to 3 minutes on high or until heated through.

STOVETOP METHOD: Transfer single portions or entire recipe to a skillet over medium-high heat. Cook, stirring, until heated through.

AMOUNT PER SERVING: Calories 340.45; Total Fat 11.71 g; Cholesterol 53.94 mg; Sodium 175.14 mg; Potassium 424.02 mg; Total Carbohydrates 33.2 g; Fiber 4.66 g; Sugar 9.86 g; Protein 26.24 g

# MOM'S GREEN CHILE CHICKEN BREASTS

One of my fondest food memories from childhood is my mom's green chile and cheese–stuffed chicken breasts. Juicy, spicy, and cheesy in every bite. Impressive as a dinner party dish, these chicken breasts can be an easy weeknight meal when kept on hand in your freezer.

**8 same-size boneless, skinless chicken breast halves**

**8 slices Monterey Jack cheese**

**8 whole green chiles from 2 cans (4 ounces, or 115 g, each)**

**2 teaspoons (12 g) Hot and Healthy Spice Blend (page 171) or salt, black pepper, and paprika to taste**

① Preheat oven to 350°F (180°C, or gas mark 4). Slice a pocket lengthwise in each chicken breast and stuff with a slice of cheese and a chile. Season the outside of the chicken breasts with Hot and Healthy Spice Blend or salt, black pepper, and paprika.

② Place chicken breasts in a large baking dish and bake for 35 minutes or until just cooked through. Let cool completely.

YIELD: 8 SERVINGS

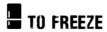 **TO FREEZE**

INDIVIDUAL SERVINGS: Wrap each breast with freezer wrap.

FOR A CROWD: Set breasts on a baking sheet, freeze until solid, and then transfer to a large freezer bag.

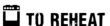 **TO REHEAT**

Let chicken thaw in the refrigerator overnight.

MICROWAVE METHOD: Reheat individual breasts on 70% power for 2 to 3 minutes or until heated through and cheese is melted.

OVEN METHOD: Preheat oven to 375°F (190°C, or gas mark 5). Place breasts in a baking dish, cover, and bake for 20 minutes or until heated through and cheese is melted.

AMOUNT PER SERVING: Calories 245.71; Total Fat 9.6 g; Cholesterol 95.68 mg; Sodium 924.07 mg; Potassium 193.2 mg; Total Carbohydrates 1.5 g; Fiber 0.47 g; Sugar 0.24 g; Protein 35.15 g

# ELEGANT AND EASY STUFFED CHICKEN BREASTS WITH WILD RICE ✗ Try

Stuffed chicken breasts are an elegant meal that is easier to prepare than it looks. Keep this dish in your freezer for nights when you crave a healthy gourmet meal or need a special quick-to-the-table dish for guests.

.....................................................................................................................................................................

**8 boneless, skinless chicken breast halves**

**4 tablespoons (90 ml) olive oil, divided**

**1 onion, finely chopped**

**1 clove garlic, crushed**

**1 cup (110 g) finely chopped sun-dried tomatoes packed in olive oil**

**1 cup (300 g) chopped marinated artichoke hearts**

**1 cup (150 g) crumbled feta**

**½ cup (30 g) chopped fresh parsley**

**2 eggs**

**2 tablespoons (28 ml) milk**

**2 cups (230 g) whole-wheat bread crumbs or Whole-Grain Bread Crumbs (page 175)**

**2 cups (320 g) wild rice**

**6 cups (1.4 L) water**

**8 ounces (225 g) sliced mushrooms**

**¼ cup (32 g) all-purpose flour**

**1 cup (235 ml) chicken broth**

**1½ cups (355 ml) low fat milk**

① Using the flat side of a mallet or a wide skillet, flatten chicken breasts between sheets of waxed paper until ¼-inch (6 mm) thick.

② Heat 1 tablespoons (14 ml) of oil in a medium skillet over medium heat. Add onion and cook, stirring often, until softened and golden. Add garlic and cook, stirring, for 30 seconds. Stir in sun-dried tomatoes, artichoke hearts, feta, and parsley. Remove from heat.

③ Divide vegetable mixture over the chicken breasts, rolling them up to hold filling. If desired, you can thread a toothpick at the seam of each roll to secure.

④ In a wide shallow dish, beat eggs with milk. Spread bread crumbs onto a large plate. Dip chicken rolls in egg, allowing excess to drip off, and then roll in crumbs, coating all sides. Refrigerate while you cook the rice.

⑤ Boil rice for 10 minutes less than package directions. Remove from heat.

⑥ Heat remaining olive oil in a large wide skillet over medium heat. Cook chicken rolls, turning occasionally, to brown all sides. Transfer to paper towels.

⑦ Add mushrooms and cook, stirring often, until mushrooms are tender and lightly browned. Sprinkle with flour, stirring to combine. Pour in chicken broth and milk and bring to a simmer. Lower heat and cook, stirring often, until thickened.

⑧ Add rice to skillet, stirring to combine. Pour rice mixture into a 13 x 9-inch (33 x 23 cm) baking dish or aluminum pan. Top with chicken rolls. Cover with foil and bake for 30 minutes or until chicken is cooked through. Cool completely.

YIELD: 8 SERVINGS

## SERVING SUGGESTION

Roasted asparagus and baby carrots elevate this meal to gourmet status. Here's how to roast asparagus: Preheat oven to 400°F (200°C, or gas mark 6). Trim bottom ends of asparagus; clean and remove green top from carrots. Toss with olive oil and spread in a layer on a rimmed baking sheet. Sprinkle with salt and freshly ground pepper; roast for 15 minutes, shaking sheet every 5 minutes to evenly brown. Vegetables are done when crisp-tender.

## 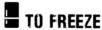 TO FREEZE

INDIVIDUAL SERVINGS: Divide chicken rolls and rice into 8 freezer- and microwave-safe containers or 1-quart (950 ml) freezer bags.

FOR A CROWD: Lay a piece of plastic wrap over chicken rolls and rice. Tightly cover dish with heavy-duty aluminum foil.

## 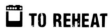 TO REHEAT

Let chicken and rice thaw in refrigerator overnight.

MICROWAVE METHOD: Reheat single portions of chicken and rice in the microwave until heated through.

OVEN METHOD: Preheat oven to 350°F (180°C, or gas mark 4). Remove plastic wrap from baking dish and re-cover with foil. Bake for 30 minutes or until heated through.

AMOUNT PER SERVING: Calories 638.22; Total Fat 21.08 g; Cholesterol 144.29 mg; Sodium 527.27 mg; Potassium 86.80 mg; Total Carbohydrates 64.64 g; Fiber 8.06 g; Sugar 6.68 g; Protein 48.27 g

# GRILLED GINGER-SESAME CHICKEN BREASTS

If it's too inclement to fire up the grill but your taste buds are craving a flame-cooked meal, sink your teeth into these Asian-inspired grilled chicken breasts. Serve them hot with Ginger and Veggie Fried Rice (page 111) or soba noodles tossed in a peanut sauce. You can also slice or dice them for salads or sandwiches.

**¼ cup (60 ml) olive oil**

**¼ cup (60 ml) tamari**

**3 tablespoons (45 ml) sesame oil**

**3 tablespoons (18 g) minced fresh ginger**

**3 cloves garlic, minced**

**Juice and zest of 2 limes**

**3 scallions, chopped (green and white parts)**

**A few grinds black pepper**

**8 small boneless skinless chicken breast halves**

① In a large plastic bag or container, whisk together oil, tamari, sesame oil, ginger, garlic, lime juice and zest, scallions, and black pepper. Place chicken in bag and marinate at least 2 hours or overnight.

② Pour marinade into a saucepan over medium-high heat. Bring to a boil for 5 minutes. Preheat grill to medium-high and oil the grate.

③ Grill chicken breasts for 5 minutes and flip. Baste the cooked side with reserved marinade. Grill for 5 more minutes or until chicken is cooked through. Baste with marinade. Remove from heat and let cool completely.

YIELD: 8 SERVINGS

---

### COOKING TIP: SERVE UP TAMARI

Tamari is a wheat-free salty-tasting condiment that is richer and more complex in flavor as well as darker and thicker than regular soy sauce. In addition, tamari is a flavorful source of antioxidants, niacin, manganese, and protein. When buying tamari, or any condiments for that matter, read the label and choose brands that are lowest in sodium and free of additives and preservatives, such as MSG.

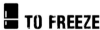 **TO FREEZE**

INDIVIDUAL SERVINGS: Wrap each chicken breast with freezer wrap.

FOR A CROWD: Place chicken breasts in one layer in a 13 x 9-inch (33 x 23 cm) aluminum baking pan. Cover tightly with aluminum foil.

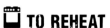 **TO REHEAT**

Let chicken thaw in the refrigerator overnight.

MICROWAVE METHOD: Reheat individual servings in the microwave on 60% power for 3 minutes or until heated through.

OVEN METHOD: Preheat oven to 350°F (180°C, or gas mark 4). Keep baking pan covered and bake chicken for 20 to 25 minutes or until heated through.

---

AMOUNT PER SERVING: Calories 187.2; Total Fat 12.61 g; Cholesterol 34 mg; Sodium 550.55 mg; Potassium 133.04 mg; Total Carbohydrates 3.48 g; Fiber 0.76 g; Sugar 0.67 g; Protein 14.8 g

# CHICKEN AND EDAMAME POT PIE

Chicken pot pie is a classic comfort food that has many tasty variations. In this rendition, edamame replaces peas while the homemade pie crust is free of trans fats and other artificial ingredients so commonly found in store-bought freezer pies.

**2 tablespoons (28 g) unsalted butter**

**2 tablespoons (28 ml) olive oil**

**1 small onion, finely chopped**

**1½ cups (195 g) diced carrots**

**1 cup (120 g) diced celery**

**2 cups (300 g) shelled edamame**

**4 cups (560 g) diced cooked skinless chicken breast**

**½ cup (63 g) all-purpose flour**

**2½ cups (570 ml) low-sodium chicken broth**

**1 cup (235 ml) half-and-half**

**Salt and freshly ground black pepper**

**1 recipe Double-Crust Whole-Wheat Pie Dough (page 204, omit sugar)**

① Preheat oven to 350°F (180°C, or gas mark 4).

② In a Dutch oven over medium heat, heat butter and oil until butter is melted, swirling pan to coat the bottom. Add onion, carrots, and celery and cook, stirring occasionally, for 7 minutes or until carrots are tender.

③ Stir in edamame and chicken. Sprinkle with flour and stir to coat. Whisk together broth and half-and-half and slowly stir into pan. Season with salt and pepper.

④ Bring mixture to a low boil and cook, stirring often, until liquid is thickened.

⑤ Roll pie dough into a 12 x 10-inch (30 x 25 cm) rectangle. Spoon chicken filling into a greased 11 x 9-inch (28 x 23 cm) casserole dish. Place dough over filling and crimp edges against the dish. Bake for 1 hour. Remove from oven and let cool completely.

YIELD: 8 SERVINGS

## NUTRITIONAL SPOTLIGHT: EDAMAME

Edamame, which are nothing more than fresh soybeans, come shelled or in fuzzy green pods and can be eaten as a snack or added to a wide variety of savory dishes. High in protein and fiber, edamame can seamlessly replace dried, fresh, or canned beans, or be tossed into any number of dishes just for the health of it.

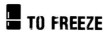 **TO FREEZE**

Place pot pie in the freezer until firm. Tightly wrap with freezer wrap.

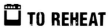 **TO REHEAT**

Let pie thaw in refrigerator overnight.

OVEN METHOD: Preheat oven to 400°F (200°C, or gas mark 6). Bake for 30 minutes or until filling is hot and crust is golden.

AMOUNT PER SERVING: Calories 272.27; Total Fat 12.69 g; Cholesterol 61.62 mg; Sodium 96.74 mg; Potassium 434.16 mg; Total Carbohydrates 15.8 g; Fiber 3.36 g; Sugar 3.03 g; Protein 23.06 g

# QUICK-FIX PAELLA

Paella is a classic Spanish comfort food boasting a mouthwatering combination of sausage, chicken, seafood, and rice. This version, featuring turkey sausage, skinless chicken thighs, and shrimp, is streamlined on fat, calories, and prep time, making it a healthy and fast dish you can have in your freezer or on your table in 30 minutes or less. This dish is best made in a paella pan, but any large wide skillet will work.

**4 cups (950 ml) reduced-sodium chicken broth**

**Pinch of saffron threads**

**3 tablespoons (45 ml) olive oil, divided**

**8 ounces (225 g) hot Italian turkey sausage, halved lengthwise, sliced crosswise**

**8 boneless, skinless chicken thighs, cubed**

**Salt and freshly ground black pepper to taste**

**1 onion, chopped**

**1 large red bell pepper, seeded, quartered, sliced**

**1 large yellow bell pepper, seeded, quartered, sliced**

**4 cloves garlic, minced**

**1 tablespoon (7 g) smoked sweet paprika**

**2 cups (460 g) paella or arborio rice**

**1 can (14.5 ounces, or 410 g) fire-roasted tomatoes or 2 cups (360 g) Fire-Roasted Tomatoes (page 39)**

**2 cups (300 g) fresh peas**

**¼ cup (15 g) chopped fresh parsley leaves**

**8 ounces (225 g) frozen medium-size shrimp, cooked**

(1) Place chicken broth in a saucepan over medium heat. Rub saffron with your fingers, crushing it, as you sprinkle it into the broth. Stir and bring to a low simmer, reducing heat to low to keep it warm.

(2) Heat 2 tablespoons (28 ml) olive oil in a paella pan or large wide skillet over medium heat. Add turkey sausage and cook, stirring often, for 2 to 3 minutes. Add chicken and cook, stirring occasionally, for 3 to 4 minutes or until chicken is lightly browned. Season with salt and pepper, stir a few more times, and then remove with a slotted spoon and set aside.

(3) Add remaining olive oil to pan and cook onions and bell pepper, stirring occasionally, until softened. Add garlic and sprinkle with paprika. Cook, stirring constantly, for 1 minute. Add rice, stirring to coat with oil and lightly toast.

(4) Add chicken broth, stirring to combine, and bring to a boil. Reduce heat to medium-low and simmer for 10 minutes, stirring occasionally.

(5) Raise heat to medium and return chicken and sausage to the pan, stirring to combine. Add tomatoes and bring to a simmer. Add more broth or water if necessary and simmer for 5 minutes.

(6) Stir in peas and parsley and simmer for 5 minutes or until rice is tender and most of the liquid has evaporated and there is a light (not burned) crust on the bottom of the mixture. Remove from heat and let cool completely. Since shrimp overcook so quickly, it's best to add them to the paella when reheating.

YIELD: 8 SERVINGS

AMOUNT PER SERVING: Calories 459; Total Fat 14.52 g; Cholesterol 123 mg; Sodium 691.21 mg; Potassium 779.14 mg; Total Carbohydrates 48.72 g; Fiber 4.91 g; Sugar 4.85 g; Protein 30.95 g

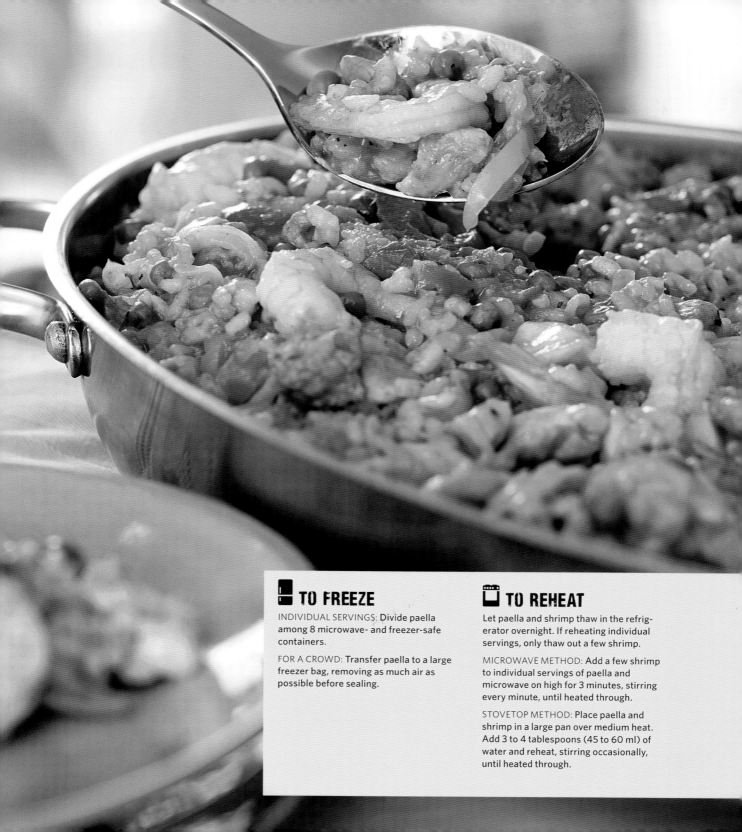

## 🧊 TO FREEZE

INDIVIDUAL SERVINGS: Divide paella among 8 microwave- and freezer-safe containers.

FOR A CROWD: Transfer paella to a large freezer bag, removing as much air as possible before sealing.

## 🔥 TO REHEAT

Let paella and shrimp thaw in the refrigerator overnight. If reheating individual servings, only thaw out a few shrimp.

MICROWAVE METHOD: Add a few shrimp to individual servings of paella and microwave on high for 3 minutes, stirring every minute, until heated through.

STOVETOP METHOD: Place paella and shrimp in a large pan over medium heat. Add 3 to 4 tablespoons (45 to 60 ml) of water and reheat, stirring occasionally, until heated through.

# ALL-OCCASION SLOPPY JANES

Sloppy Joes have nothing on this healthy, ground turkey Sloppy Jane version. Fun for the whole family, when you have company, or simply want a comforting meal midday, you can bake these to hot, juicy perfection while you steam vegetables, make a salad, or prep dessert.

16 whole-wheat sandwich buns or Honey Whole-Wheat Freezer Rolls (page 129), split

1 tablespoon (15 ml) canola oil

1 pound (455 g) lean chicken sausage

1 pound (455 g) lean ground turkey

1 medium onion, chopped

3 cloves garlic, minced

1 cup (150 g) dried currants

1 cup (100 g) coarsely chopped unsalted roasted almonds

2 tablespoons (32 g) tomato paste

16 ounces (455 g) tomato sauce

1 tablespoon (15 ml) balsamic vinegar

1 teaspoon dried oregano

½ teaspoon salt

Freshly ground black pepper to taste

① Remove the centers from the tops and bottoms of the buns. Set shells aside and cover to keep fresh. Place bread crumbs in a bowl.

② In a large saucepan, heat oil over medium-high heat. Cook sausage, ground turkey, and onion, stirring often, until sausage is browned. Add garlic, currants, and almonds and cook, stirring often, for 2 minutes. Stir in reserved bread crumbs.

③ Stir in tomato paste. Add tomato sauce, vinegar, oregano, salt, and pepper. Bring to a simmer and then reduce heat to medium-low. Simmer for 10 minutes. Remove from heat and let cool completely.

④ Fill the bottoms of the buns with meat mixture. Cover with tops of buns.

YIELD: 16 SERVINGS

## SERVING SUGGESTIONS

Serve these sloppy, savory goodies with any of these vegetable sides:

- Quick and Snappy Beans with Hazelnuts (page 100)
- Naturally Sweet Agave-Glazed Carrots (page 101)
- Fast-Fix Zucchini Slaw (page 102)
- Tender Roasted Vegetables (page 105)
- Fast and Fabulous Fava Beans (page 106)

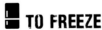 **TO FREEZE**

Place on a baking sheet and freeze until firm. Tightly wrap with freezer wrap and place in 1-gallon (3.8 L) freezer bags.

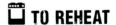 **TO REHEAT**

OVEN METHOD: Preheat oven to 350°F (180°C, or gas mark 4). Unwrap and place on a baking sheet. Bake for 35 to 40 minutes or until heated through and buns are toasty.

AMOUNT PER SERVING: Calories 305.6; Total Fat 13.6 g; Cholesterol 56.59 mg; Sodium 828.68 mg; Potassium 470.06 mg; Total Carbohydrates 32.79 g; Fiber 3.77 g; Sugar 11.8 g; Protein 15.46 g

# VEGGIE-LICIOUS TURKEY BURRITOS

Shredded carrots and tomato sauce give the tasty turkey filling the texture of pulled beef or pork without the calories or fat. Lima beans are a nice addition of high-fiber vegetable protein.

2 tablespoons (28 ml) canola oil

1 onion, halved, thinly sliced

1 pound (455 g) lean ground turkey breast

Salt and freshly ground black pepper to taste

3 cups (330 g) shredded carrots

1 cup (145 g) golden raisins

1 can (15 ounces, or 425 g) tomato sauce

1 teaspoon rubbed dried sage

1 teaspoon ground cinnamon

3 tablespoons (12 g) finely chopped fresh parsley

2 cups (200 g) lima beans

1½ cups (225 g) crumbled queso blanco cheese

10 whole-wheat flour tortillas

① Heat oil in a large pot over medium-high heat. Cook onion and ground turkey, stirring often, for 5 to 6 minutes or until turkey is browned and onion is softened. Season with salt and pepper. Stir in shredded carrots and cook, stirring often, for 3 minutes.

② Add raisins, tomato sauce, sage, cinnamon, parsley, and lima beans, stirring to combine. Cook for 2 minutes and then reduce heat to medium-low and simmer for 5 minutes, stirring occasionally. Remove from heat and let cool completely.

③ Divide turkey mixture among tortillas and sprinkle with cheese. Fold tortilla ends over and roll burrito-style.

YIELD: 10 BURRITOS, OR 10 SERVINGS

## TO FREEZE

INDIVIDUAL SERVINGS: Wrap each burrito with freezer wrap and place in a large freezer bag.

FOR A CROWD: Place burritos on a baking sheet and freeze until solid. Set in an aluminum quarter-sheet (12 x 8-inch, or 30 x 20 cm) cake pan and cover with freezer wrap.

## TO REHEAT

Let burritos thaw in refrigerator overnight.

MICROWAVE METHOD: Reheat individual burritos on high for 1½ minutes or until heated through.

OVEN METHOD: Preheat oven to 350°F (180°C, or gas mark 4). Remove freezer wrap from baking pan and bake for 15 to 20 minutes or until heated through.

AMOUNT PER SERVING: Calories 304.74; Total Fat 11.6 g; Cholesterol 44.47 mg; Sodium 671.31 mg; Potassium 593.88 mg; Total Carbohydrates 35.57 g; Fiber 11.85 g; Sugar 15.32 g; Protein 15.94 g

# RED QUINOA GRAIN SALAD

Quinoa, a protein-rich grain, comes in red, black, or ivory colors, giving you a medley of hues to use for this flavorful dish. Serve it warm in the winter or as a cool grain salad in the summer when you need to beat the heat. This also makes a great one-dish meal for campouts or picnics.

1½ cups (260 g) red quinoa

3 cups (700 ml) low-sodium chicken broth

2 tablespoons (28 ml) olive oil

1 onion, finely chopped

3 carrots, thinly sliced

1 pound (455 g) sliced mushrooms

2 cloves garlic, minced

Juice of 1 lemon

1¼ pounds (570 g) sweet turkey sausage, diced  *optional*

¼ cup (24 g) finely chopped fresh mint

1 cup (160 g) dried cherries

3 tablespoons (45 ml) raspberry vinaigrette, store-bought or homemade (see recipe)

Salt and freshly ground black pepper

4 ounces (115 g) crumbled feta cheese

① In a medium saucepan, bring quinoa and broth to a boil. Reduce heat to low, cover, and cook for 15 minutes or until broth is absorbed. Remove from heat.

② Heat oil in a large saucepot over medium heat. Add onion and carrots and cook, stirring often, for 4 minutes. Add mushrooms and cook, stirring often, for 5 minutes. Add garlic and cook, stirring, for 1 minute.

③ Add lemon juice and sausage and cook, stirring occasionally, until sausage is lightly browned. Stir in quinoa, mint, cherries, and vinaigrette and cook for 2 minutes. Season with salt and pepper. Remove from heat and let cool completely. Stir in feta.

YIELD: 8 SERVINGS

## BONUS RECIPE: RASPBERRY VINAIGRETTE

- 1 pint (455 g) fresh raspberries
- 1 tablespoon (20 g) agave or honey
- 1 tablespoon (11 g) Dijon mustard
- Juice from half a lemon
- 2 teaspoons grated lemon zest
- 2 teaspoons fresh thyme leaves
- 2 tablespoons (28 ml) red wine vinegar
- ⅔ cup (160 ml) extra-virgin olive oil
- Salt and freshly ground black pepper to taste

Purée first 7 ingredients. With machine running, add olive oil until blended. Season with salt and pepper.

AMOUNT PER SERVING: Calories 581.32; Total Fat 33.22 g; Cholesterol 65.73 mg; Sodium 659.47 mg; Potassium 861.07 mg; Total Carbohydrates 50.67 g; Fiber 8.57 g; Sugar 6.92 g; Protein 25.21 g

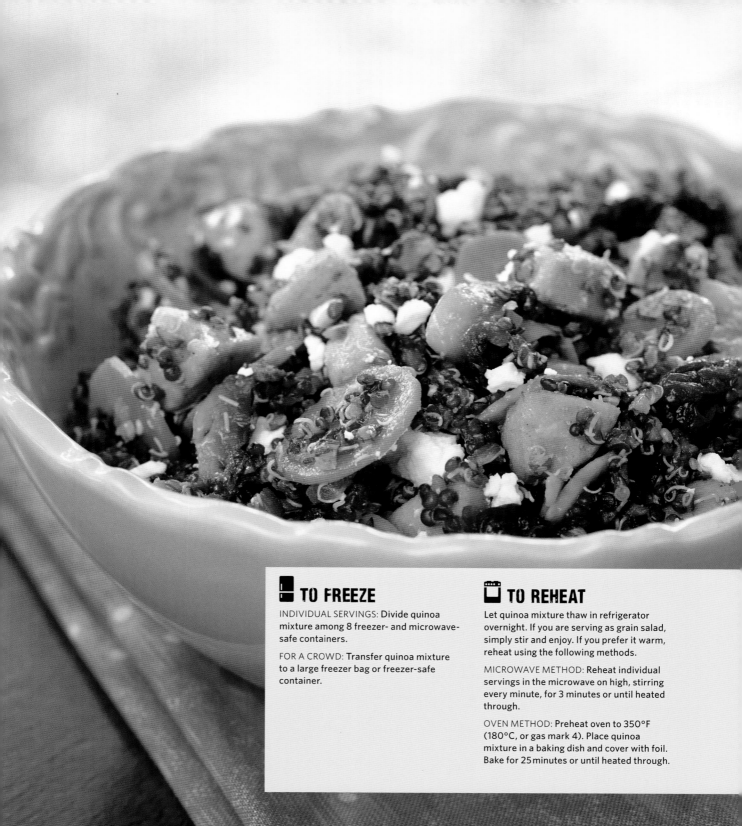

## 🗄 TO FREEZE

INDIVIDUAL SERVINGS: Divide quinoa mixture among 8 freezer- and microwave-safe containers.

FOR A CROWD: Transfer quinoa mixture to a large freezer bag or freezer-safe container.

## 🍳 TO REHEAT

Let quinoa mixture thaw in refrigerator overnight. If you are serving as grain salad, simply stir and enjoy. If you prefer it warm, reheat using the following methods.

MICROWAVE METHOD: Reheat individual servings in the microwave on high, stirring every minute, for 3 minutes or until heated through.

OVEN METHOD: Preheat oven to 350°F (180°C, or gas mark 4). Place quinoa mixture in a baking dish and cover with foil. Bake for 25 minutes or until heated through.

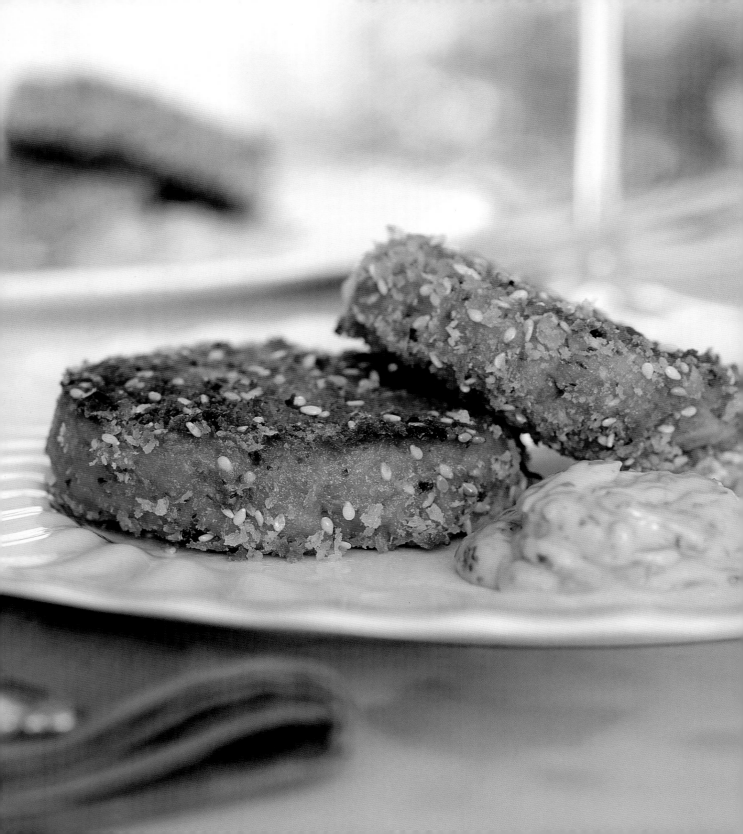

# ASIAN-SPICED TUNA CAKES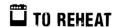

Rich in heart-healthy and brain-boosting omega-3s and a super source of lean protein, these Asian-style tuna cakes can be on the table in minutes and pair perfectly with a leafy green salad. Serve with your favorite seafood sauce or try the Creamy Wasabi Sauce (recipe below).

**3 cans (6 ounces, or 170 g) albacore tuna packed in water, flaked**

**3 cups (150 g) panko, divided**

**½ cup thinly sliced scallions (green and white parts)**

**¼ cup (25 g) chopped fresh cilantro**

**3 tablespoons (18 g) finely chopped fresh ginger**

**1 clove garlic, minced**

**Juice and grated zest of 1 lime**

**4 eggs, lightly beaten**

**1 tablespoon (15 ml) sesame oil**

**2 tablespoons (28 ml) tamari**

**2 tablespoons (28 ml) rice wine vinegar**

**1 tablespoon (13 g) granulated sugar**

**½ cup (72 g) sesame seeds**

① In a food processor, combine tuna, 1 cup (50 g) panko, scallions, cilantro, ginger, garlic, and lime juice and zest. Pulse to coarsely chop.

② Add eggs, sesame oil, tamari, vinegar, and sugar. Process until well-combined. Shape tuna mixture into 16 cakes.

③ Combine remaining panko and sesame seeds in a shallow dish. Coat tuna cakes with panko mixture.

YIELD: 16 CAKES, OR 8 SERVINGS

## BONUS RECIPE: CREAMY WASABI SAUCE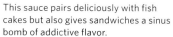

This sauce pairs deliciously with fish cakes but also gives sandwiches a sinus bomb of addictive flavor.

- 2 cups (450 g) light mayonnaise
- 2 cloves garlic, minced
- ¼ cup (4 g) finely chopped cilantro
- 2 teaspoons (23 ml) toasted sesame oil
- 1½ tablespoons (24 g) wasabi paste (or to taste)

Whisk together ingredients, adjusting to taste.

## TO FREEZE

Arrange tuna cakes on a baking sheet and freeze until solid. Wrap each cake in freezer wrap and transfer to 1-gallon (3.8 L) freezer bags, removing as much air as possible before sealing.

## TO REHEAT

Thaw tuna cakes in the refrigerator overnight.

STOVETOP METHOD: Heat 2 to 3 tablespoons (28 to 45 ml) canola or peanut oil in a large skillet over medium heat. Cover skillet and cook tuna cakes for 4 minutes per side or until heated through and lightly browned. Drain on paper towels.

OVEN METHOD: Preheat broiler. Place tuna cakes on a baking sheet and broil for 6 to 8 minutes or until heated through and lightly browned. Bake for 25 minutes or until heated through.

AMOUNT PER SERVING: Calories 713.65; Total Fat 56.12 g; Cholesterol 171.92 mg; Sodium 1585.97 mg; Potassium 420.67 mg; Total Carbohydrates 31.87 g; Fiber 2.66 g; Sugar 8.15 g; Protein 23.88 g

# AGAVE-GLAZED GRILLED SALMON STEAKS

Loaded with omega-3s and succulently glazed with agave, grilled salmon pairs deliciously with Quick and Snappy Beans with Hazelnuts (page 100), Oven-Baked Hush Puppies (page 109), or the salad below.

.................................................................................................................................................

¼ cup (60 g) firmly packed brown sugar

¼ cup (60 g) agave syrup

2 tablespoons (32 g) Dijon mustard

½ cup (120 ml) white wine

2 cloves garlic, minced

1 tablespoon (6 g) minced fresh ginger

3 tablespoons (12 g) finely chopped fresh parsley

1 teaspoon salt

½ teaspoon ground white pepper

8 salmon fillets (6 ounces, or 170 g, each)

① In a medium bowl, whisk together sugar, agave, mustard, wine, garlic, ginger, parsley, salt, and pepper. Pour into a large plastic bag and add fish. Refrigerate for 2 to 3 hours.

② Preheat grill to medium-high. Pour marinade in a saucepan over medium-high heat and boil for 5 minutes. Grill fish for 3 to 4 minutes, flip, and baste cooked side with glaze from saucepan. Grill 3 to 4 minutes, flip, and baste again. Salmon is done when it flakes when pressed with the back of a fork. Remove from heat and cool completely.

YIELD: 8 SERVINGS

## BONUS RECIPE: CHERRY, MINT, AND FETA SALAD

- 3 cups (465 g) pitted cherries, halved
- 3 tablespoons (18 g) finely chopped mint or more to taste
- 3 tablespoons (30 g) minced red onion
- ⅓ cup (50 g) crumbled feta
- 2 teaspoons balsamic vinegar
- 1 tablespoon (28 ml) olive oil
- Salt and freshly ground black pepper to taste

Toss all ingredients in a bowl. Serve as is or on top of a bed of spinach or mixed salad greens.

 ## TO FREEZE

INDIVIDUAL SERVINGS: Place each steak in a freezer- and microwave-safe container.

FOR A CROWD: Place fish on a baking sheet and freeze until solid. Place in a large freezer bag, removing as much air as possible before sealing.

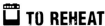 ## TO REHEAT

Let fish thaw in refrigerator overnight.

MICROWAVE METHOD: Reheat individual servings on 70% power for 2 to 3 minutes or until heated through. Don't overcook.

OVEN METHOD: Preheat oven to 400°F (200°C, or gas mark 6). Place desired number of steaks in a baking pan and cover with foil. Bake for 10 to 15 minutes or until fish is heated through.

AMOUNT PER SERVING: Calories: 427.05; Total Fat 21.2 g, Cholesterol 107.16 mg, Sodium 445.32 mg, Potassium 693.26 mg, Total Carbohydrates 16.66 g, Fiber 0.73 g, Sugar 15.04 g, Protein 37.91 g,

# SHRIMP-STUFFED PORTOBELLOS

Seasoned shrimp filling piled in meaty portobellos makes this recipe an unusual but deliciously filling dish. For a change, you can swap out the jumbo mushrooms for button or cremini and serve as a tasty little appetizer.

## FOR THE SHRIMP STUFFING:

**10 ounces (280 g) reduced-fat butter crackers**

**6 tablespoons (24 g) finely chopped fresh parsley**

**3 tablespoons (45 ml) olive oil**

**½ cup (80 g) finely chopped onion**

**6 tablespoons (38 g) finely chopped celery**

**½ cup (55 g) grated carrot**

**½ cup (75 g) finely chopped red bell pepper**

**Salt and freshly ground black pepper to taste**

**2 cloves garlic, minced**

**8 ounces (225 g) cooked chopped shrimp**

**2 teaspoons Old Bay Seasoning**

**2 tablespoons (28 ml) dry sherry**

**1 tablespoon (15 ml) Worcestershire sauce**

**1 cup (235 ml) clam juice or water**

## FOR THE MUSHROOMS:

**8 portobello mushrooms, stems and gills removed**

**Olive oil**

**Salt and freshly ground black pepper to taste**

① Preheat oven to 425°F (220°C, or gas mark 7). Place crackers in a plastic bag and crush with a rolling pin. Add parsley, shaking to combine, and set aside.

② Heat oil in a large skillet over medium heat and cook onion, celery, carrot, and bell pepper, stirring often, until softened. Season with salt and pepper. Add garlic and cook, stirring, for 1 minute more. Add shrimp, Old Bay, sherry, Worcestershire, and clam juice or water, stirring to combine, and remove from heat. Cool completely.

③ Rub mushrooms with olive oil. Season with salt and pepper. Place on a baking sheet and roast for 10 to 12 minutes or until softened. Set aside to cool completely. Stuff mushrooms with shrimp stuffing and set on a baking sheet.

YIELD: 8 SERVINGS

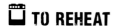

## TO FREEZE

INDIVIDUAL SERVINGS: Place mushrooms in the freezer until solid. Wrap individually with freezer wrap and place in 1 or 2 large freezer bags.

FOR A CROWD: Place mushrooms in the freezer until solid. Transfer mushrooms to a freezer container or freezer bag, layering with waxed paper, if necessary.

## TO REHEAT

Let mushrooms thaw in the refrigerator for a few hours or overnight.

MICROWAVE METHOD: Individual servings can be reheated in the microwave but won't have a crisp crust that oven baking and broiling provide. To reheat, microwave mushrooms on high for 2 minutes or until heated through.

OVEN METHOD: Preheat oven to 350°F (180°C, or gas mark 4). Place mushrooms on a baking sheet and bake for 15 minutes. Turn broiler on and broil until stuffing is lightly browned and crisped.

AMOUNT PER SERVING: Calories 727.44; Total Fat 12.53 g; Cholesterol 43.13 mg; Sodium 3816.25 mg; Potassium 1729.02 mg; Total Carbohydrates 134.93 g; Fiber 6.71 g; Sugar 36.1 g; Protein 17.91 g

# SUSTAINABLE SWORDFISH AND PINEAPPLE KABOBS

Long considered an eco-worst choice of seafood, swordfish from Canada, Hawaii, and some other U.S. locations is now considered a "best choice" (avoid imported varieties). Salmon and tuna steaks are juicy alternatives if sustainable swordfish is unavailable. Serve kabobs with Apricot Pistachio Rice Pilaf (page 113) and Quick and Snappy Beans with Hazelnuts (page 100).

⅓ cup (80 ml) olive oil

½ cup (120 ml) pineapple juice

½ cup (20 g) fresh basil

3 cloves garlic

Zest and juice of 1 orange

½ teaspoon salt

¼ teaspoon freshly ground black pepper

2 tablespoons (28 ml) white wine vinegar

2 tablespoons (40 g) honey

2 pounds (900 g) swordfish steaks, cut into 24 cubes

24 large cubes fresh pineapple

8 wooden skewers, soaked in water for 30 minutes

① In a food processor, combine oil, pineapple juice, basil, garlic, orange zest and juice, salt, pepper, vinegar, and honey. Transfer to a large plastic bag and add fish. Refrigerate for 2 to 3 hours.

② Preheat grill to medium-high. Thread swordfish and pineapple onto skewers. Oil grill grate and grill kabobs for 3 to 4 minutes per side or until just medium-rare. Remove from grill and allow to cool completely.

YIELD: 8 SKEWERS, OR 8 SERVINGS

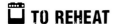 **TO FREEZE**

Place kabobs on a baking sheet and freeze until solid. Transfer to a heavy-duty freezer-safe container (skewers may puncture plastic bags) and seal.

**TO REHEAT**

Let kabobs thaw in refrigerator overnight.

MICROWAVE METHOD: Place kabobs on a microwave-safe plate and microwave on high for 2 to 3 minutes or until heated through. Don't overcook the fish.

OVEN METHOD: Preheat broiler. Place kabobs on a baking sheet or broil pan and broil for 2 to 3 minutes, turn, and continue to broil for 1 to 2 minutes or until heated through.

## COOKING TIP: CUT PINEAPPLE WITH CARE

Here's how to prepare fresh pineapple: Lay pineapple sideways on a cutting board. Using a sharp knife, remove the green top. Cut off the top and bottom of pineapple. Turn pineapple upright and cut skin from the flesh following the curve of the fruit. Use the knife tip or the tip of a peeler to remove any remaining bits of skin. Cut pineapple crosswise into slices. Use a paring knife to cut out the core of each of the slices.

AMOUNT PER SERVING: Calories 487.86; Total Fat 14.12 g; Cholesterol 44.36 mg; Sodium 253.82 mg; Potassium 912.99 mg; Total Carbohydrates 70.94 g; Fiber 7.53 g; Sugar 51.51 g; Protein 25.52 g

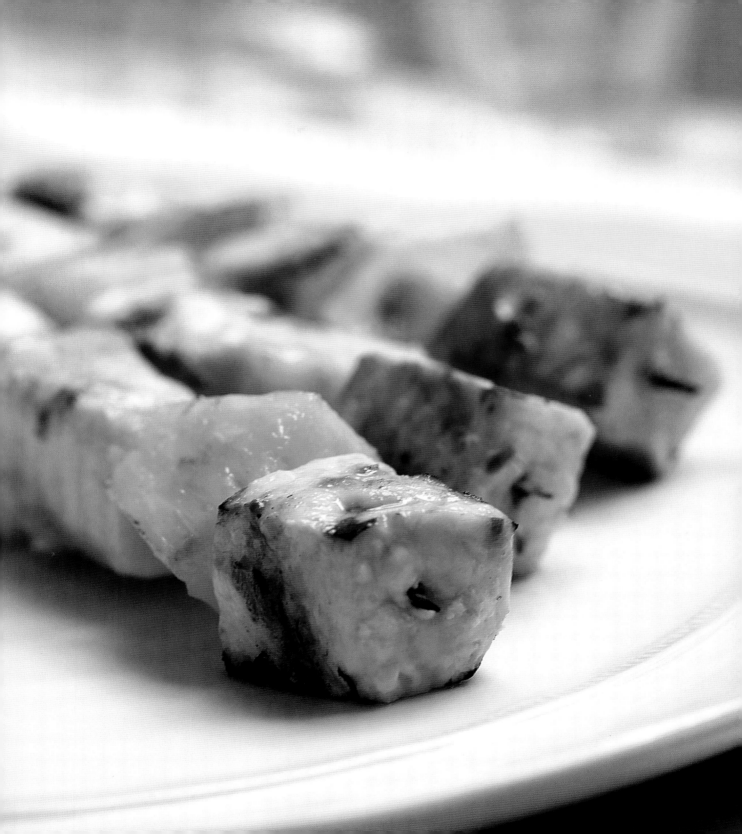

# CHAPTER 5

# SOUPS, STEWS, AND CHILIS
## HEAVENLY, HEALING, STEAMING MEDLEYS

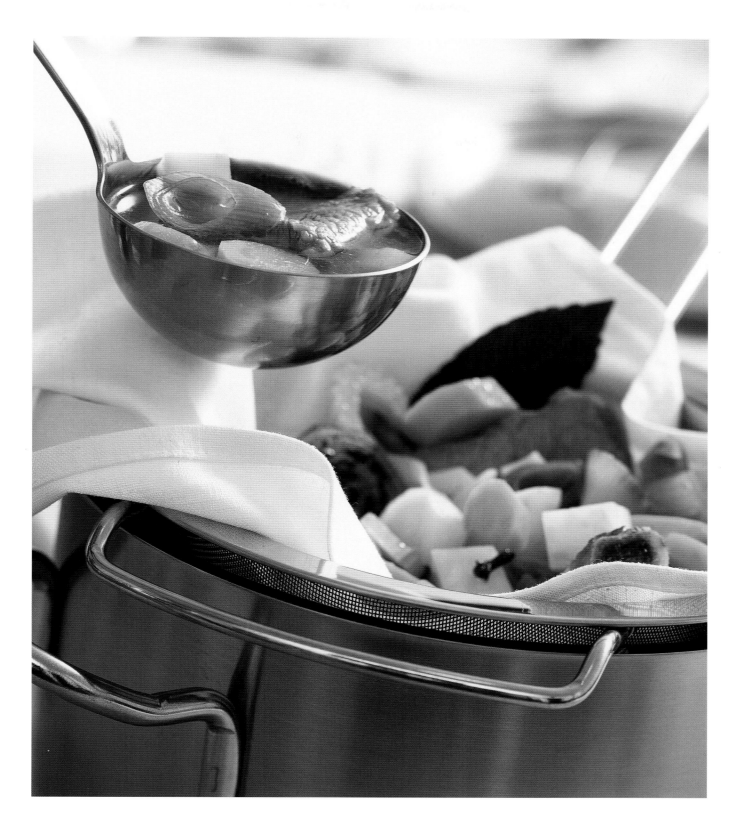

# GAZPACHO WITH VEGETABLES GALORE

Chilled soup hits the spot in the summer swelter when cooking is out of the question but you need a healthy meal. This gazpacho is one of the healthiest low-calorie soups you can sip. Chock-full of nutrient-rich tomatoes, vegetables, and herbs, pair it with a slice of Zesty Garlic-Rosemary Bread (page 126).

6 vine-ripened tomatoes, cored, chopped

5 cups (1.2 L) spicy vegetable juice

2 cucumbers, peeled, seeded, chopped

1 red onion, chopped

1 green bell pepper, seeded, chopped

1 jalapeño, halved, seeded, finely chopped

1 bunch watercress

⅓ cup (80 ml) red wine vinegar

2 tablespoons (28 ml) extra-virgin olive oil

3 tablespoons (3 g) chopped fresh cilantro

1 clove garlic, minced

Salt and freshly ground black pepper to taste

① In a large bowl, combine all ingredients in a food processor and pulse to purée to desired consistency. Gazpacho can be smooth or a bit chunky.

YIELD: 12 CUPS (2.8 L), OR 12 SERVINGS

### NUTRITION TIP: EAT MORE SOUP

Having a low-calorie soup, whether warm or chilled, as a first course for a meal can reduce the total amount of calories you consume in that meal because the soup fills you up before the main meal hits the table. However, don't expect the same results from cream-based chowders or soups loaded with high-fat meats; soups such as gazpacho and broth-based soups work because they are low in calories.

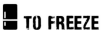 TO FREEZE

INDIVIDUAL SERVINGS: Pour gazpacho into twelve (8-ounce, or 235 ml) plastic freezer jars.

FOR A CROWD: Pour gazpacho into a 1-gallon (3.8 L) freezer bag, lay bag flat in a casserole dish, and freeze until solid. Remove casserole dish.

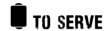 TO SERVE

Thaw overnight in the refrigerator. Stir a few times and serve chilled.

AMOUNT PER SERVING: Calories 64.69; Total Fat 2.5 g; Cholesterol 0 mg; Sodium 309.55 mg; Potassium 461.58 mg; Total Carbohydrates 9.93 g; Fiber 2.42 g; Sugar 6.15 g; Protein 1.83 g

*Try this (or variation) for Xmas holidays 2013*

# GARDEN TOMATO BASIL SOUP

When the crisp fall weather starts to set in, harvest those late-summer tomatoes and transform them into a warm tomato soup. Richly flavored with onions, garlic, and basil, serve this heart-healthy soup as a starter course or pair with a salad for a light lunch or dinner. Garnish with crumbled feta cheese, chopped hard-cooked egg, or a swirl of crème fraiche.

⅓ cup (80 ml) olive oil

3 cups (480 g) thinly sliced onions

4 cloves garlic, minced

3½ pounds (1.6 kg) garden fresh tomatoes, halved, seeded, chopped

8 cups (1.9 L) vegetable broth

Grated zest and juice of 1 lemon

Generous pinch of brown sugar

1 cup (40 g) chopped fresh basil

① In a large saucepan over medium-low heat, heat olive oil.

② Add onions and cook, stirring occasionally, until soft and golden, about 15 minutes. Add garlic and cook, stirring, for 1 minute.

③ Add tomatoes, broth, lemon zest and juice, and sugar. Increase heat to medium-high and bring to a boil. Reduce heat to medium-low and simmer for 20 minutes. Stir in basil and remove from heat.

④ Transfer soup to a food processor or blender and in batches, purée soup. You may also use an immersion stick blender to purée in the saucepan. Let soup cool completely.

YIELD: 5 QUARTS (4.7 L), OR 20 SERVINGS

## SERVING SUGGESTION

Add a salad to this soup for a more substantial and healthier meal. One of my favorites is spinach, toasted almonds, sliced radishes, currants, and a balsamic vinaigrette.

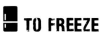 **TO FREEZE**

INDIVIDUAL SERVINGS: Ladle soup into freezer- and microwave-safe containers.

FOR A CROWD: Divide soup between two 1-gallon (3.8 L) freezer bags, lay bags flat in a baking dish, and freeze until solid. Remove baking dish.

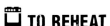 **TO REHEAT**

Let soup thaw in refrigerator overnight. Serve it chilled or warm.

MICROWAVE METHOD: Reheat individual servings of soup in the microwave at 60% power for 2 minutes or until heated through.

STOVETOP METHOD: Reheat soup in a saucepan over medium heat for 10 to 15 minutes or until heated through.

AMOUNT PER SERVING:  Calories 124.02; Total Fat 5.41 g; Cholesterol 0.99 mg; Sodium 658.32 mg; Potassium 395.93 mg; Total Carbohydrates 16.8 g; Fiber 2.95 g; Sugar 3.16 g; Protein 3.52 g

# CHICKEN, VEGETABLE, AND WILD RICE SOUP

Chicken and wild rice are a delectable pair in this hearty belly-warming soup. For the best flavor, visit your farmers' market to pick the freshest, most nutrient-packed vegetables.

3 tablespoons (45 ml) olive oil

1 pound (455 g) boneless, skinless chicken breast, cut into bite-size pieces

2 large leeks, white part only, thinly sliced crosswise

2 stalks celery, finely chopped

2 carrots, chopped

8 ounces (225 g) sliced mushrooms

2 cloves garlic, minced

6 cups (1.4 L) low-sodium chicken broth

½ cup (120 ml) sherry

2 tablespoons (5 g) fresh thyme leaves

1 bay leaf

1½ cups (248 g) cooked wild rice

Salt and freshly ground black pepper to taste

① Heat oil in a large pot over medium-high heat. Cook chicken, stirring often, until cooked through. With a slotted spoon, transfer chicken to a plate to keep warm.

② Add leeks, celery, carrots, and mushrooms to the pot and cook, stirring often, until leeks are soft and mushrooms release their juices. Add garlic and cook, stirring, for 1 minute.

③ Add chicken broth, sherry, thyme, bay leaf, and reserved chicken (and any juices that collected on the plate) and bring to a simmer. Reduce heat to low and simmer for 10 minutes. Add rice and simmer for 10 more minutes. Season with salt and pepper and remove from heat to cool completely.

YIELD: 14 CUPS (3.3 L), OR 7 SERVINGS

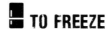 TO FREEZE

INDIVIDUAL SERVINGS: Transfer soup to freezer- and microwave-safe containers.

FOR A CROWD: Transfer soup to a 1-gallon (3.8 L) freezer bag and lay flat in a baking dish. Freeze until solid and then remove baking dish.

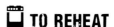 TO REHEAT

Let soup thaw in the refrigerator overnight.

MICROWAVE METHOD: Reheat soup in the microwave on high for 2 to 3 minutes or until heated through.

STOVETOP METHOD: Reheat soup in a large pot over medium-high heat, stirring occasionally, until heated through.

AMOUNT PER SERVING: Calories 345.94; Total Fat 8.34 g; Cholesterol 38.98 mg; Sodium 142.62 mg; Potassium 683.68 mg; Total Carbohydrates 38.09 g; Fiber 3.95 g; Sugar 4.08 g; Protein 26.64 g

# LEAN AND LUSCIOUS LAMB STEW

Lamb stew is wholesome comfort in a bowl. This succulent mélange of lamb, vegetables, dried plums, almonds, and sherry will have your family beyond happy to gather around the dinner table to warm their bones after a long winter day. Serve with egg noodles or new potatoes.

2 tablespoons (28 ml) olive oil

2 pounds (900 g) lean boneless lamb, cut into bite-size pieces

1 onion, chopped

2 carrots, chopped

2 stalks celery, chopped

3 cloves garlic, minced

1 tablespoon (2 g) rosemary

1 tablespoon (7 g) smoked paprika

½ cup (48 g) raw almonds, finely ground

1 cup (175 g) chopped dried plums

1 bay leaf

1 cup (235 ml) sherry

3 cups (700 ml) vegetable broth

Salt and freshly ground black pepper to taste

Sour cream or crème fraiche for serving (optional)

① Heat oil in a Dutch oven over medium-high heat. Add lamb and cook, stirring often, until browned on all sides. With a slotted spoon, transfer lamb to a plate.

② Add onion, carrots, and celery, and cook, stirring often, until onion is translucent and carrots are just tender. Stir in garlic, rosemary, and paprika, cooking for 1 minute.

③ Sprinkle with ground almonds, stirring to coat. Add dried plums, bay leaf, sherry, and broth and bring to a boil. Reduce heat to low and simmer, covered, for 30 minutes. Remove lid, stir, and season with salt and pepper. Continue to simmer for 15 minutes. Remove from heat and remove the bay leaf. Cool completely.

YIELD: 10 CUPS (2.4 L), OR 8 SERVINGS

## NUTRITION SPOTLIGHT: LAMB

Lamb is a delicious meat that is high in tryptophan, selenium, zinc, and vitamin B-12 while being a great source of protein. One 4-ounce (115 g) serving of lamb provides over 100% of the daily value for tryptophan, an amino acid associated with appetite regulation, quality sleep, and improved mood. Like other meats, choose the leaner cuts of lamb, such as leg of lamb, loin chops, and lamb shoulder, to avoid the extra saturated fat and calories.

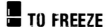 TO FREEZE

INDIVIDUAL SERVINGS: Divide stew into freezer- and microwave-safe containers.

FOR A CROWD: Transfer stew to a 1-gallon (3.8 L) freezer bag. Lay flat in a baking dish and freeze until solid. Remove baking dish.

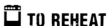 TO REHEAT

Let stew thaw in the refrigerator overnight.

MICROWAVE METHOD: Reheat individual portions in the microwave on 60% power for 3 to 4 minutes or until heated through. Stir in sour cream or crème fraiche before serving.

STOVETOP METHOD: Reheat stew in a saucepan over medium-high heat, stirring occasionally, for 10 to 15 minutes or until heated through. Remove from heat and stir in sour cream or crème fraiche.

AMOUNT PER SERVING: Calories 449.56; Total Fat 24.24 g; Cholesterol 76 mg; Sodium 703.57 mg; Potassium 775.28 mg; Total Carbohydrates 25.42 g; Fiber 4.21 g; Sugar 2.15 g; Protein 25.32 g

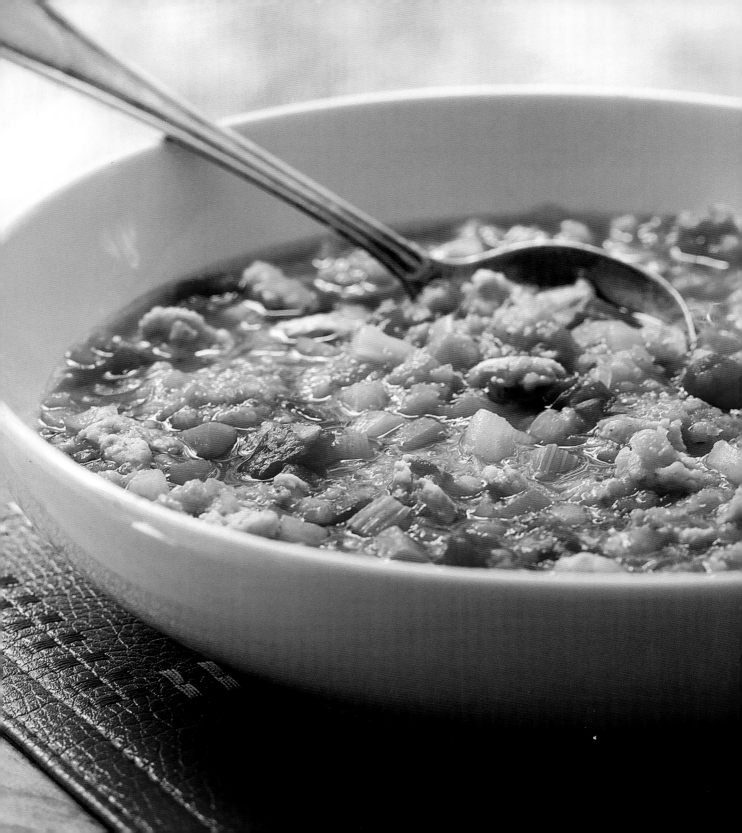

# HEARTY RED LENTIL STEW

Red lentils are not only easier to prepare than other types of beans, but they are also an excellent source fiber, protein, folic acid, molybdenum, and other essential vitamins and minerals. Their pretty red hue also makes this stew a stunner at the table. For a colorful change, try green, yellow, or black lentils.

2 cups (384 g) red lentils, rinsed, picked over

3 cups (700 ml) water

1 tablespoon (15 ml) olive oil

1¼ pounds (570 g) sweet Italian turkey sausage, casings removed, crumbled 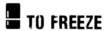 *optional*

2 onions, chopped

2 carrots, chopped

1 stalk celery, chopped

2 teaspoons fresh thyme

2 teaspoons minced fresh rosemary

1 can (14.5 ounces, or 410 g) fire-roasted diced tomatoes, or 2 cups (360 g ) Fire-Roasted Tomatoes (page 39)

1 bay leaf

8 cups (1.9 L) vegetable broth

① In a pot over medium-high heat, stir together lentils and water. Bring to a boil and then reduce heat, cover pot, and simmer for 15 to 20 minutes or until lentils are very soft. Drain and set aside.

② In a Dutch oven over medium-high heat, heat olive oil. Cook sausage, stirring often, until browned. Remove from pan and drain on paper towels. Add onion, carrots, and celery and cook, stirring often, until softened, about 7 minutes.

③ Stir in thyme, rosemary, and tomatoes. Cook, stirring occasionally, for 3 minutes. Add lentils, sausage, bay leaf, and broth and bring to a boil. Reduce heat to medium-low and simmer for 45 minutes. Remove bay leaf. Let stew cool completely.

YIELD: 12 CUPS (2.8 L), OR 12 SERVINGS

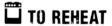 TO FREEZE

INDIVIDUAL SERVINGS: Transfer stew to freezer- and microwave-safe containers.

FOR A CROWD: Transfer stew to one or two 1-gallon (3.8 L) freezer bags, lay flat in a baking dish, and freeze until solid. Remove baking dish.

TO REHEAT

Let stew thaw overnight in the refrigerator.

MICROWAVE METHOD: Individual servings of stew can be reheated in the microwave on high for 2 to 3 minutes or until heated through.

STOVETOP METHOD: Reheat stew in a saucepan over medium-high heat, stirring occasionally, for 15 minutes or until heated through.

AMOUNT PER SERVING: Calories 376.99; Total Fat 13.67 g; Cholesterol 39.28 mg; Sodium 1421.43 mg; Potassium 704.11 mg; Total Carbohydrates 44.82 g; Fiber 7.77 g; Sugar 3.61 g; Protein 19.8 g

# WILD DUCK AND TURKEY SAUSAGE GUMBO

Gumbo is a Cajun-inspired mélange of meat or seafood (or both) and rice with many mouthwatering variations depending on where it is made. This recipe features duck and sausage, making it a rich-flavored stew that is culinary biss upon first bite. If desired, add sliced fresh okra when you add the onions.

.......................................................................................................................................................

**¼ cup (60 ml) canola oil**

**1 wild duck (3 to 4 pounds, or 1.4 to 1.8 kg), skin removed, cut up**

**⅓ cup (42 g) all-purpose flour**

**8 ounces (225 g) smoked turkey sausage, sliced**

**1 onion, chopped**

**1 green bell pepper, chopped**

**2 stalks celery, sliced**

**1 tablespoon (4 g) minced fresh parsley**

**2 cloves garlic, minced**

**1 can (14.5 ounces, or 410 g) fire-roasted diced tomatoes, or 2 cups (360 g) Fire-Roasted Tomatoes (page 39)**

**1 bay leaf**

**1 tablespoon (15 ml) Worcestershire sauce**

**1 tablespoon (4 g) finely chopped fresh tarragon**

**Salt and freshly ground black pepper to taste**

**4 cups (950 ml) water**

**4 cups (660 g) Family-Favorite Freezer Rice (page 110)**

① Heat oil in a Dutch oven over medium heat and add duck, turning often, until browned. Use tongs to remove and set aside.

② Add flour to drippings and cook, stirring often for 10 to 12 minutes or until roux is a medium brown. Add sausage, onion, green pepper, celery, parsley, and garlic and cook, stirring often, for 10 minutes.

③ Add tomatoes, bay leaf, Worcestershire sauce, tarragon, and salt and pepper, stirring to combine. Stir in duck and water and bring to a boil. Reduce heat to a low simmer, cover, and simmer for 1 hour or until duck is tender.

④ Remove duck from the bones. Cut duck meat into bite-size pieces and then add back to pan. Simmer for 5 minutes or until heated through. Remove bay leaf and allow gumbo to cool completely.

YIELD: 8 SERVINGS

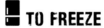 ## TO FREEZE

INDIVIDUAL SERVINGS: Divide gumbo into 8 microwave- and freezer-safe containers.

FOR A CROWD: Transfer gumbo to a large freezer bag, seal, and lay flat in a casserole dish. Freeze until solid and then remove casserole dish.

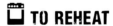 ## TO REHEAT

Let gumbo and rice thaw in the refrigerator overnight.

MICROWAVE METHOD: Reheat individual servings of gumbo and rice in the microwave for 2 to 3 minutes or until heated through.

STOVETOP METHOD: Reheat gumbo in a large saucepan or Dutch oven over medium heat, stirring often, until heated through. Reheat rice in a large saucepan over medium heat with 2 to 3 tablespoons (28 to 45 ml) of water, stirring often, until heated through.

AMOUNT PER SERVING: Calories 555.22; Total Fat 36.45 g; Cholesterol 158.73 mg; Sodium 583.61 mg; Potassium 1022.9 mg; Total Carbohydrates 18.03 g; Fiber 2.96 g; Sugar 7.28 g; Protein 36.22 g

# CROWD-PLEASING CARAMELIZED ONION SOUP

Onion soup topped with toasted bread and melted cheese is the perfect midday winter eat and a delectable starter course for more substantial evening meals. Low in calories yet laden with flavor, onions make a mouthwatering base for this soup, especially when caramelized so their natural sweetness exudes forth.

3 tablespoons (42 g) unsalted butter

3 tablespoons (45 ml) olive oil

6 cups (960 g) finely sliced onions

Salt and freshly ground black pepper to taste

1 tablespoon (13 g) granulated sugar

1 tablespoon (15 ml) cider vinegar

3 tablespoons (24 g) all-purpose flour

8 cups (1.9 L) vegetable broth or, for a richer flavor, beef broth

2 bay leaves

Croutons or thin slices of French bread, toasted

Shredded Gruyère cheese

1  In a Dutch oven over medium heat, stir butter and oil together until butter is melted. Add onions and cook, stirring occasionally, until soft and golden, about 10 minutes. Season with salt and pepper.

2  Stir in sugar and vinegar and cook, stirring often, until onions are caramelized and lightly browned.

3  Sprinkle flour over onions and stir for 2 minutes. Stir in broth and bay leaves. Bring soup to a low boil. Reduce heat to medium-low and simmer for 30 minutes. Adjust seasoning with salt and pepper. Remove bay leaves and allow soup to cool completely.

YIELD: 8 CUPS (1.9 L), OR 8 SERVINGS

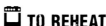 ## TO FREEZE

INDIVIDUAL SERVINGS: Ladle soup into freezer- and microwave-safe containers.

FOR A CROWD: Transfer soup to a 1-gallon (3.8 L) freezer bag, lay flat in a baking dish, and freeze until solid. Remove baking dish.

 ## TO REHEAT

Thaw soup in refrigerator overnight.

MICROWAVE METHOD: Reheat individual servings in the microwave on high for 2 minutes or until heated through. Garnish with croutons and shredded Gruyère cheese.

OVEN METHOD: Preheat broiler. Reheat soup in a saucepan over medium-high heat, stirring occasionally, until heated through. Transfer to ovenproof mugs. Float croutons or a thin slice of toasted French bread on soup and sprinkle with grated Gruyère. Place mugs on a baking sheet and place under the broiler until cheese is melted and bubbly.

AMOUNT PER SERVING:  Calories 311.1; Total Fat 13.38 g; Cholesterol 13.75 mg; Sodium 1631.7 mg; Potassium 567.52 mg; Total Carbohydrates 41.49 g; Fiber 5.32 g; Sugar 6.73 g; Protein 7.63 g

# CURRIED WINTER SQUASH SOUP

Curry meets sweet with this satisfying winter squash treat. Loaded with vitamins A and C, potassium, and fiber, winter squash becomes a silky soup emanating warm and spicy flavors. Serve swirled with a dollop of honey Greek yogurt and garnished with finely chopped cilantro for a pretty contrast in color.

**4 pounds (1.8 kg) acorn or butternut squash**

**3 tablespoons (45 ml) olive oil**

**2 onions, chopped**

**2 cloves garlic, minced**

**2 tablespoons (12 g) minced fresh peeled ginger**

**1 tablespoon (6.3 g) curry powder**

**1 teaspoon ground coriander**

**3 cups (705 ml) half-and-half or milk**

**Salt and freshly ground black pepper to taste**

① Preheat oven to 375°F (190°C, or gas mark 5). Poke holes in squash and place in baking dish or on a rimmed baking sheet. Bake for 45 minutes or until squash is tender. Set aside until cool enough to handle.

② Cut squash in half and remove seeds. Spoon flesh into a food processor or blender.

③ Heat oil in a large skillet over medium-high heat. Add onions and cook, stirring often, until soft and golden, about 10 minutes. Add garlic and ginger and cook, stirring often, for 1 minute. Sprinkle with curry and coriander, stirring to coat.

④ Transfer onion mixture to the food processor or blender. Add 1 cup (235 ml) half-and-half or milk and purée. Blend in remaining half-and-half or milk. Season with salt and pepper. Let cool completely.

YIELD: 10 CUPS (2.4 L), OR 8 SERVINGS

## NUTRITION TIP: EAT YOUR COLORS

The more colorful your fruits and vegetables, the more nutrient-dense your meals. Winter squash, with its brilliant yellow and orange flesh, is loaded with nutrients, such as antioxidants, fiber, and powerful phytochemicals that promote the health of your heart, eyes, bones, and digestive and immune systems while combating cancer and aiding in wound healing. When planning your family's meals, reach for recipes featuring the richest, darkest fruits and vegetables.

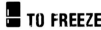 ## TO FREEZE

INDIVIDUAL SERVINGS: Transfer soup to freezer- and microwave-safe containers.

FOR A CROWD: Place soup in a 1-gallon (3.8 L) freezer bag, lay flat in a baking dish, and freeze until solid. Remove baking dish.

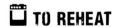 ## TO REHEAT

Let soup thaw overnight in the refrigerator.

MICROWAVE METHOD: Reheat individual portions of soup in the microwave for 3 to 4 minutes, stirring every minute, until heated through.

STOVETOP METHOD: Transfer soup to a saucepan over medium heat and cook, stirring occasionally, for 10 minutes or until soup is heated through.

AMOUNT PER SERVING: Calories 281.6; Total Fat 15.92 g; Cholesterol 33.35 mg; Sodium 48.09 mg; Potassium 978.09 mg; Total Carbohydrates 34.13 g; Fiber 5.42 g; Sugar 6.44 g; Protein 5.46 g

# VENISON BLACK BEAN CHILI

Black beans lend their nutrient-dense, rich flavor to this wild game stew. A lean, highly prized meat, venison is a stellar source of vitamin B12 and other B vitamins. If venison is unavailable, simply substitute a lean cut of beef. To serve, top with crumbled goat cheese, chopped fresh cilantro, and jalapeño slices.

**2 tablespoons (28 ml) canola oil**

**½ pound (227 g) spicy Italian turkey sausage, casings removed, crumbled**

**2 cups (320 g) chopped onion**

**5 cloves garlic, minced**

**1½ pounds (680 g) boneless venison loin, trimmed and cut into ½-inch (1.3 cm) pieces**

**¼ cup (65 g) tomato paste**

**6 cups (1.4 L) reduced-sodium vegetable broth**

**2 cups (360 g) chopped Roma tomatoes**

**3 tablespoons (24 g) ancho chile powder**

**1 teaspoon kosher salt**

**1½ teaspoons (3.8 g) ground cumin**

**1 teaspoon ground coriander**

**2 cans (15 ounces, or 425 g, each) no-salt-added black beans, rinsed and drained**

① Heat oil a large Dutch oven over medium-high heat. Add sausage, onion, and garlic and cook, stirring occasionally, for 6 minutes or until onion is tender.

② Add venison and cook, stirring often, for 4 minutes or until venison is browned. Stir in tomato paste and cook for 3 minutes, stirring occasionally.

③ Add vegetable broth, tomatoes, chile powder, cumin, and coriander, scraping bottom of pan to loosen browned bits. Bring to a boil, cover, reduce heat to medium-low, and simmer for 1 hour or until venison is tender. Stir in black beans and cook 10 minutes more. Remove from heat and cool.

YIELD: 8 SERVINGS

## COOKING TIP: COOK SLOW AND LOW

The slow cooker is one of the best timesaving kitchen appliances. Sure, the microwave can quickly reheat cooked meals, but it doesn't come close to achieving the depth and complexity of flavors from stove cooking or slow cooking. This chili, along with any of the hot soups and stews in this book, can be cooked in a slow cooker, saving you time so you can either batch cook other dishes or take care of that to-do list.

 **TO FREEZE**

INDIVIDUAL SERVINGS: Transfer completely cooled chili to freezer- and microwave-safe containers and freeze.

FOR A CROWD: Transfer completely cooled chili to 1-gallon (3.8 L) freezer bags. Seal and lay bags in a baking dish. Freeze solid and then remove baking dish and stack bags.

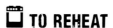 **TO REHEAT**

Let chili thaw in refrigerator overnight.

MICROWAVE METHOD: Heat individual portions of chili on high for 3 to 4 minutes.

STOVETOP METHOD: Heat chili in a saucepan over medium heat, stirring occasionally, until hot.

AMOUNT PER SERVING: Calories 335.88; Total Fat 11.81 g; Cholesterol 34.45 mg; Sodium 1474.95 mg; Potassium 620.38 mg; Total Carbohydrates 30.09 g; Fiber 5.41 g; Sugar 4.11 g; Protein 29.34 g

# PORK AND POBLANO POZOLE

One of my favorite stews, pozole is a mouthwatering mélange of pork, hominy, chiles, garlic, and Mexican spices. Filling yet far from fattening, this rendition will healthfully warm your winter evenings.

2 tablespoons (28 ml) vegetable oil

1 onion, coarsely chopped

4 cloves garlic, minced

1½ pounds (680 g) boneless pork loin, cut into bite-size cubes

1½ teaspoons ground cumin

1 teaspoon ground coriander

1 teaspoon dried oregano

1 teaspoon sweet paprika

Salt and freshly ground black pepper to taste

4 poblano chiles, roasted, peeled, seeded, diced

1 jalapeño, seeded, minced

4 cups (950 ml) reduced-sodium vegetable broth

1 can (28 ounces, or 785 g) hominy, drained

① Heat oil in a large pot over medium heat. Add onion and cook, stirring often, for 4 to 5 minutes. Add garlic and cook, stirring for 30 seconds. Add pork, cumin, coriander, oregano, paprika, and salt and pepper and cook, stirring occasionally, until pork is browned on all sides.

② Stir in poblanos and jalapeño. Add enough vegetable broth to cover ingredients with 2 inches (5 cm) of liquid. Stir and bring to a boil. Lower heat and simmer for 30 to 40 minutes. Stir in hominy and simmer for 20 minutes more. Remove from heat and allow to cool completely.

YIELD: 8 SERVINGS

## SERVING SUGGESTIONS

Garnish this hearty stew with diced avocado, shredded cheese, and a sprinkle of finely chopped cilantro. If you're craving a side dish, try a bowl of baked tortilla chips and a fruity salsa—the crunch from the chips and sweet from the salsa lend a delectable contrast to the spicy stew.

 TO FREEZE

INDIVIDUAL SERVINGS: Divide soup into 8 freezer- and microwave-safe containers and freeze.

FOR A CROWD: Transfer soup to a 1-gallon (3.8 L) freezer bag and lay flat in a baking dish. Freeze until solid, and then remove baking dish.

 TO REHEAT

Let soup thaw in the refrigerator overnight.

MICROWAVE METHOD: Reheat individual portions of soup on 60% power for 3 to 4 minutes or until heated through.

STOVETOP METHOD: Reheat soup in a large saucepan over medium-high heat, stirring occasionally, until heated through.

AMOUNT PER SERVING: Calories 503.2; Total Fat 7.75 g; Cholesterol 56.1 mg; Sodium 172.51 mg; Potassium 534.32 mg; Total Carbohydrates 81.43 g; Fiber 5.54 g; Sugar 1.88 g; Protein 28.01 g

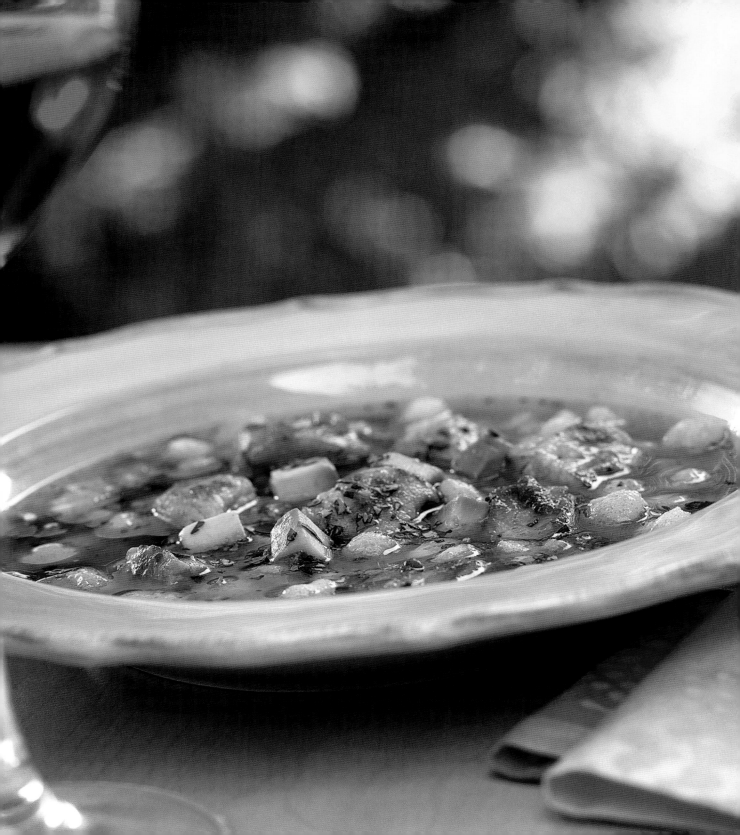

# HOT AND SPICY CHICKEN CORN CHOWDER

I created my first homemade corn chowder the first winter I lived in Montana. Coming from the sunny central coast of California, the below-freezing temperatures and powdery snow led me straight to the kitchen to cook up soups that quickly and thoroughly warmed my bones. Since then, I've created many variations on this quintessential cold-weather meal. This recipe boasts colorful vegetables and tongue-tantalizing textures that satisfy whether for a substantial lunch or a light supper.

**4 cups (616 g) fresh corn kernels, divided**

**1½ cups (355 ml) half-and-half**

**2½ cups (570 ml) milk**

**1 tablespoon (15 ml) olive oil**

**1 pound (455 g) spicy low-fat chicken sausage, halved, sliced**

**1 cup (110 g) sun-dried tomatoes packed in olive oil, chopped**

**2 carrots, finely chopped**

**3 shallots, minced**

**Grated zest and juice of 1 lime**

**2 cloves garlic, minced**

**2 cans (4 ounces, or 115 g, each) diced mild green chiles**

**1 tablespoon (4 g) fresh oregano**

**3 tablespoons (3 g) finely chopped fresh cilantro**

**Salt and freshly ground black pepper to taste**

① Purée 2½ cups (385 g) corn kernels with half-and-half. In a stockpot over medium heat, combine corn mixture and milk and bring to a low simmer. Reduce heat if necessary.

② Heat oil in a large skillet over medium heat and cook sausage, stirring often, until browned. Using a slotted spoon, transfer to a plate. Add tomatoes and carrots and cook, stirring often, until carrots are just tender. Add shallots and cook, stirring often, until softened. Add lime zest, juice, and garlic and cook, stirring, for 1 minute.

③ Add remaining corn, sausage, vegetable mixture, chiles, oregano, and cilantro to stockpot, stirring to combine. Bring to a low simmer (do not boil) and simmer for 5 minutes. Season with salt and pepper. Remove from heat and cool completely.

YIELD: 10 SERVINGS

 **TO FREEZE**

INDIVIDUAL SERVINGS: Divide chowder among 10 freezer- and microwave-safe containers.

FOR A CROWD: Transfer chowder to a large freezer bag, seal, and lay flat in a baking dish. Freeze until solid and then remove baking dish.

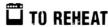 **TO REHEAT**

Let chowder thaw in the refrigerator for a few hours.

MICROWAVE METHOD: Gently reheat individual servings in the microwave on 50% power, stirring every minute, for 3 minutes or until heated through. Do not boil.

STOVETOP METHOD: In a stockpot over medium heat, bring chowder to a low simmer, stirring often, until heated through. Do not boil.

AMOUNT PER SERVING: Calories 347.42; Total Fat 11.15 g; Cholesterol 25.64 mg; Sodium 339.74 mg; Potassium 1332.09 mg; Total Carbohydrates 56.51 g; Fiber 9.41 g; Sugar 15.07 g; Protein 12.92 g

# THREE-BEAN ITALIAN MINESTRONE SOUP

Warm and wonderful, this high-fiber soup is a delightful reward after a long day of snow play. Serve with Honey Whole-Wheat Freezer Rolls (page 129). For a vegetarian change, simply omit the turkey sausage and add an extra can of kidney or cannellini beans. The pasta is also optional, if you prefer a lower-carb version of the soup.

3 tablespoons (45 ml) olive oil

1 pound (455 g) sweet Italian turkey sausage, casings removed, crumbled

1 onion, chopped

3 stalks celery, finely chopped

4 carrots, diced

3 cloves garlic, minced

8 ounces (225 g) cremini mushrooms, sliced

3 cans (14.5 ounces, or 410 g, each) crushed tomatoes

3 cups (700 ml) low-sodium vegetable broth

1 tablespoon (6 g) dried Italian seasoning

1 pound (455 g) fresh green beans, ends trimmed, snapped into 1-to-2-inch (2.5-to-5 cm) pieces

1 can (15 ounces, or 425 g) cannellini beans, rinsed, drained

1 can (15 ounces, or 425 g) kidney beans, rinsed, drained

Salt and freshly ground black pepper to taste

2 cups (210 g) whole-wheat elbow macaroni (optional)

Shaved Parmesan cheese

① Heat olive oil in a stockpot over medium heat. Add sausage and cook, stirring often, until lightly browned. Use a slotted spoon to transfer it to a plate.

② Add onion, celery, and carrots and cook, stirring often, until vegetables are just soft. Stir in garlic and mushrooms and cook, stirring often, until mushrooms release their liquid. Add tomatoes, broth, Italian seasoning, beans, and sausage, stirring to combine. Bring to a simmer and season with salt and pepper.

③ If you are adding pasta, cook it in boiling salted water for 1 minute less than package directions. Pasta should be toothsome, not mushy soft. Drain and add to soup. Remove from heat and allow soup to cool completely.

YIELD: 8 SERVINGS

## NUTRITION SPOTLIGHT: BEANS

Beans are an ultra-economical, super versatile source of protein, fiber, iron, folate, and other vitamins and minerals. There is an ample variety of dry and canned beans that you can conveniently add to soups, stews, grain salads, pasta dishes, and more. Like fruits and vegetables, the richer the color of the bean, the healthier. Black beans are one of the best sources of antioxidants, but any of the beans and legumes will provide a dietary boon to your health.

 **TO FREEZE**

INDIVIDUAL SERVINGS: Divide soup among 8 freezer- and microwave-safe containers. Stir in a sprinkling of Parmesan and seal.

FOR A CROWD: Transfer soup to a large freezer bag, seal, and lay flat in a baking dish. Freeze until solid and then remove baking dish.

 **TO REHEAT**

Let soup thaw in refrigerator overnight.

MICROWAVE METHOD: Individual servings of soup can be reheated in the microwave on high, stirring every minute, for 2 to 3 minutes or until heated through.

STOVETOP METHOD: Pour soup into a stockpot over medium-high heat. Reheat, stirring occasionally, until heated through. Divide into serving bowls and serve sprinkled with Parmesan cheese.

AMOUNT PER SERVING: Calories 423.74; Total Fat 11.64 g; Cholesterol 34.64 mg; Sodium 953.95 mg; Potassium 1010.14 mg; Total Carbohydrates 61.64 g; Fiber 14.6 g; Sugar 4.7 g; Protein 24.42 g

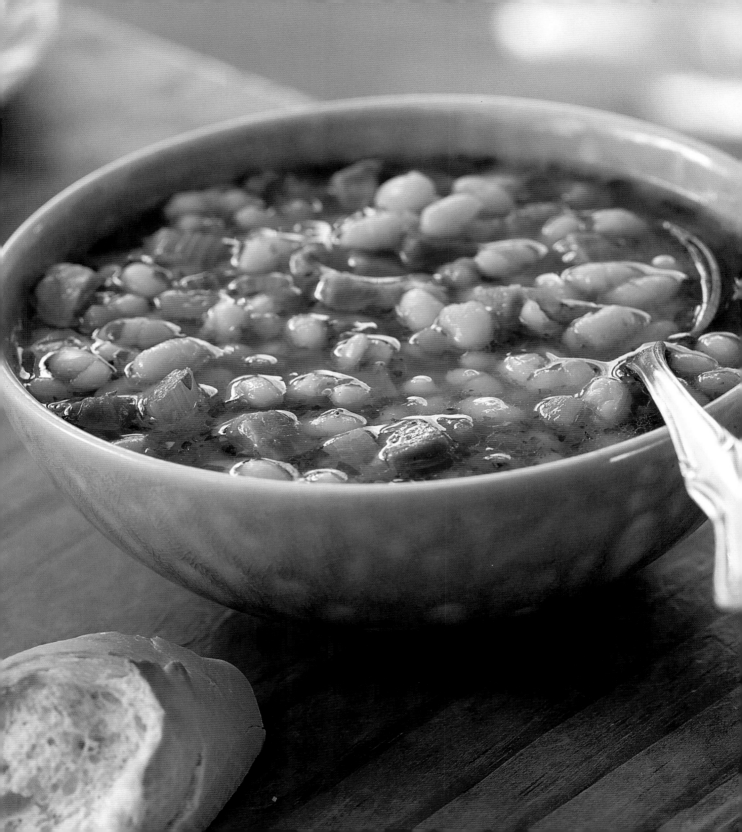

# HEALTHY SMOKED HAM AND BEAN SOUP

Adding beans to any soup elevates its nutritiousness while stretching your food budget dollars. Adding a ham hock to the simmer gives this soup a delectable depth of smoky flavor. Try this soup with a wedge of Fast and Easy Fresh Herb Focaccia (page 137) or a slice of Whole-Grain Seeded Bread (page 128).

**2 tablespoons (28 ml) canola oil**

**1 onion, diced**

**1 carrot, diced**

**2 stalks celery, diced**

**3 cloves garlic, minced**

**1 sprig fresh rosemary**

**¼ cup (15 g) chopped fresh parsley**

**1 dried bay leaf**

**1 teaspoon dried oregano**

**1 tablespoon (56 g) fennel seeds**

**1 pound (455 g) ham steak, fat removed, diced**

**1 smoked ham hock**

**1 pound (455 g) dried small white beans, rinsed and picked through**

**8 cups (1.9 L) water, plus extra if needed**

**Salt and freshly ground black pepper to taste**

① Heat oil in a stockpot over medium heat. Add onion, carrot, and celery and cook, stirring occasionally, for 10 to 15 minutes or until onion is translucent and carrots are softened.

② Add garlic, rosemary, parsley, bay leaf, oregano, and fennel to the pot. Cook, stirring often, for 2 to 3 minutes.

③ Add ham steak, ham hock, and beans. Cover ingredients with 8 cups (1.9 L) of water, stirring to combine. Season with salt and pepper. Increase heat to high and bring soup to a boil.

④ Reduce heat to medium-low and simmer for 2 hours or until beans are tender. Add water, ¼ cup (60 ml) at a time, if soup starts to get too thick, stirring after each addition. Remove the ham hock and rosemary sprig. Set aside to cool completely.

YIELD: 8 SERVINGS

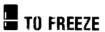 ## TO FREEZE

INDIVIDUAL SERVINGS: Transfer soup to single-serving freezer- and microwave-safe containers.

FOR A CROWD: Transfer soup to 1-gallon (3.8 L) freezer bags. Lay bags on their side in a baking dish and freeze. Remove baking dish and stack bags in freezer.

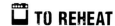 ## TO REHEAT

Let soup defrost in the refrigerator overnight.

MICROWAVE METHOD: Reheat individual servings of soup on high for 3 to 4 minutes.

STOVETOP METHOD: Place soup in a saucepan over medium heat. Simmer, stirring occasionally, for 10 minutes or until heated through.

AMOUNT PER SERVING:  Calories 186.01; Total Fat 6.95 g; Cholesterol 29.34mg; Sodium 813.08 mg; Potassium 1335.22 mg; Total Carbohydrates 38.16 g; Fiber 9.86 g; Sugar 1.43 g; Protein 25.88 g

# CHAPTER 6

## SIDE DISHES AND VEGETARIAN OPTIONS

### EAT AND ENJOY YOUR VEGGIES

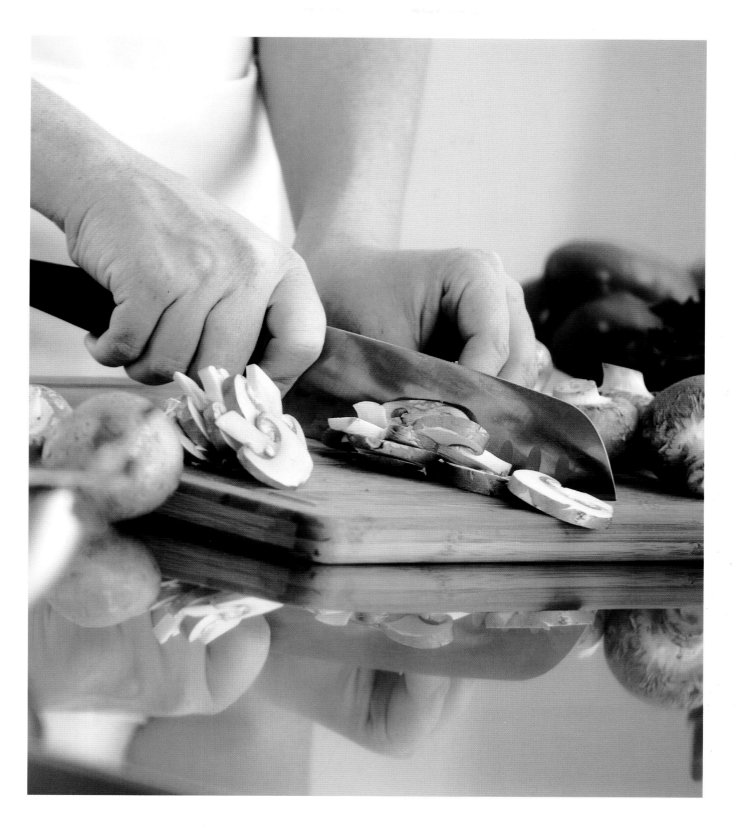

# QUICK AND SNAPPY BEANS WITH HAZELNUTS

Plain green beans get a flavorful gourmet update with the addition of hazelnuts, ginger, and hazelnut oil. Hazelnuts add crunch and a delicious dose of healthy fats and vitamin E while ginger lends its vibrant zing.

**1 cup (135 g) whole hazelnuts**

**2 pounds (900 g) fresh snap beans, ends trimmed, cut diagonally in half**

**1 tablespoon (15 ml) hazelnut oil**

**2 tablespoons (28 ml) canola oil**

**1 tablespoon (6 g) minced fresh peeled ginger**

**1 clove garlic, minced**

**Salt and freshly ground black pepper to taste**

① Preheat oven to 350°F (180°C, or gas mark 4). Place hazelnuts in a pie tin and place in the oven. Cook for 10 minutes, shaking pan occasionally, until nuts are toasted. Place nuts in a kitchen towel and rub vigorously to remove the skins. Coarsely chop and set aside to cool completely.

② In a large pot of boiling salted water, cook beans for 2 minutes to blanch. Drain and place in an ice bath to halt the cooking. Drain and pat dry with a towel.

③ In a large skillet over medium heat, heat oils. Add ginger and garlic and cook, stirring often, for 1 to 2 minutes. Add the beans and cook, stirring often, for 3 minutes. Remove from the heat and let cool completely.

YIELD: 8 SERVINGS

## NUTRITION SPOTLIGHT: HAZELNUTS

Hazelnuts contain nearly 75% monounsaturated fat and less than 4% saturated fat, making them a tasty heart-healthy nibble; research shows that hazelnuts can lower blood pressure and decrease cholesterol. Hazelnuts are also a yummy source of vitamin E, magnesium, folate, calcium, iron, B vitamins, fiber, and phytochemicals associated with a decreased risk of heart disease, cancer, depression, urinary tract infections, and because of the folate a reduced risk of neural tube defects.

## TO FREEZE

Place nuts in a 1-quart (946 ml) freezer bag, removing as much air as possible before sealing.

INDIVIDUAL SERVINGS: Divide beans into freezer- and microwave-safe containers or 1-quart (950 ml) freezer bags, removing as much as possible before sealing.

FOR A CROWD: Place beans in a 1-gallon (3.8 L) freezer bag, removing as much as possible before sealing.

## TO REHEAT

Let nuts and beans thaw in the refrigerator overnight.

MICROWAVE METHOD: For individual servings, sprinkle nuts over beans, toss to coat, loosely cover, and reheat on high for 2 minutes or until heated through.

STOVETOP METHOD: Place beans in a skillet over medium-high heat. Sprinkle with nuts and cook, stirring often, until beans are heated through.

AMOUNT PER SERVING: Calories 197.18; Total Fat 16.41 g; Cholesterol 0 mg; Sodium 6.97 mg; Potassium 378.47 mg; Total Carbohydrates 11.53 g; Fiber 5.58 g; Sugar 2.49 g; Protein 4.83 g

# NATURALLY SWEET AGAVE-GLAZED CARROTS

Carrot sticks may be a healthy nibble, but oftentimes the family's picky eaters don't have a penchant to snack on them. Glazing them in agave and orange juice not only tenderizes them but also gives them a sweet flavor that turns them to palate-pleasing instead of picked over.

........................................................................................................................................................

**2 pounds (900 g) carrots, cut into batons**

**¼ cup (60 ml) water**

**¼ cup (60 ml) freshly squeezed orange juice**

**3 tablespoons (42 g) unsalted butter, melted**

**2 tablespoons (40 g) agave nectar**

**3 tablespoons (7 g) fresh lemon thyme leaves**

**Salt and freshly ground black pepper to taste**

① In a large skillet over medium heat, combine carrots, water, and orange juice. Cover and cook, stirring occasionally, until carrots are just tender.

② Add butter, agave, and thyme and cook, uncovered, stirring often, until liquid has evaporated and carrots are glazed. Season with salt and pepper, stirring one last time. Remove from heat and let cool completely.

YIELD: 8 SERVINGS

## COOKING TIP: SWEETEN IT UP NATURALLY WITH AGAVE

Agave is a low-glycemic natural sweetener with a consistency similar to honey. It can replace sugar and honey in most recipes. When replacing sugar with agave, remember the following tips:

- Use about ⅓ cup (107 g) of agave nectar for every 1 cup (200 g) of sugar.
- Reduce the liquid ingredients in recipes by one-third.
- Reduce your oven temperature by 25°F (4°C).
- In recipes calling for honey, you can substitute equal portions.

 **TO FREEZE**

INDIVIDUAL SERVINGS: Place carrots in freezer- and microwave-safe containers.

FOR A CROWD: Place carrots in a 1-gallon (3.8 L) freezer bag, removing as much air as possible before sealing.

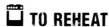 **TO REHEAT**

Let carrots thaw in the refrigerator for a few hours.

MICROWAVE METHOD: Reheat individual servings on high for 2 minutes or until heated through.

STOVETOP METHOD: Reheat carrots in a skillet over medium heat, stirring occasionally, for 5 minutes or until heated through.

AMOUNT PER SERVING: Calories 102.99; Total Fat 4.56 g; Cholesterol 11.29 mg; Sodium 79.22 mg; Potassium 386.31 mg; Total Carbohydrates 15.74 g; Fiber 3.56 g; Sugar 9.63 g; Protein 1.21 g

# FAST-FIX ZUCCHINI SLAW

Cabbage isn't the only star of the slaws. Zucchini is another low-calorie choice that can be tossed with herbs, spices, and a tangy dressing as a side for burgers or grilled meals as well as a welcome topping for sandwiches or filling for wraps.

**6 large zucchini, ends trimmed, coarsely grated or cut into matchsticks**

**½ cup (30 g) finely chopped fresh parsley**

**½ cup (32 g) chopped fresh dill**

**1 tablespoon (6 g) fennel seeds** *optional*

**1 cup (150 g) dried currants**

**2 tablespoons (28 ml) white wine vinegar**

**1 tablespoon (11 g) Dijon mustard**

**⅓ cup (80 ml) extra-virgin olive oil**

**Salt and freshly ground black pepper to taste**

① In a large bowl, combine zucchini, parsley, dill, fennel, and currants.

② In a small bowl, whisk together vinegar, mustard, and olive oil. Pour over zucchini and toss to coat. Season with salt and pepper.

YIELD: 10 CUPS (1.5 KG), OR 15 SERVINGS

---

### COOKING TIP: TURN UP THE SLAW HEAT
For a tongue-tantalizing change, you can add sweet or spice to this simple slaw recipe by doing one or more of the following:
- Replace part of the zucchini with shredded daikon radish.
- Substitute cilantro for the dill and omit the fennel seeds.
- Add 1 jalapeño, seeded (if desired) and minced.
- Replace 1 tablespoon (15 ml) olive oil for chili oil.
- Add 1 tablespoon (20 g) agave or honey.

---

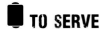 **TO FREEZE**

INDIVIDUAL SERVINGS: Place slaw in freezer- and microwave-safe containers or 1-quart (950 ml) freezer bags.

FOR A CROWD: Place slaw in a 1-gallon (3.8 L) freezer bag, removing as much air as possible before sealing.

**TO SERVE**

Let slaw thaw in the refrigerator.

---

AMOUNT PER SERVING: Calories 49.69; Total Fat 0.79 g; Cholesterol 0 mg; Sodium 24.36 mg; Potassium 342.01 mg; Total Carbohydrates 10.83 g; Fiber 1.88 g; Sugar 8.17 g; Protein 1.65 g

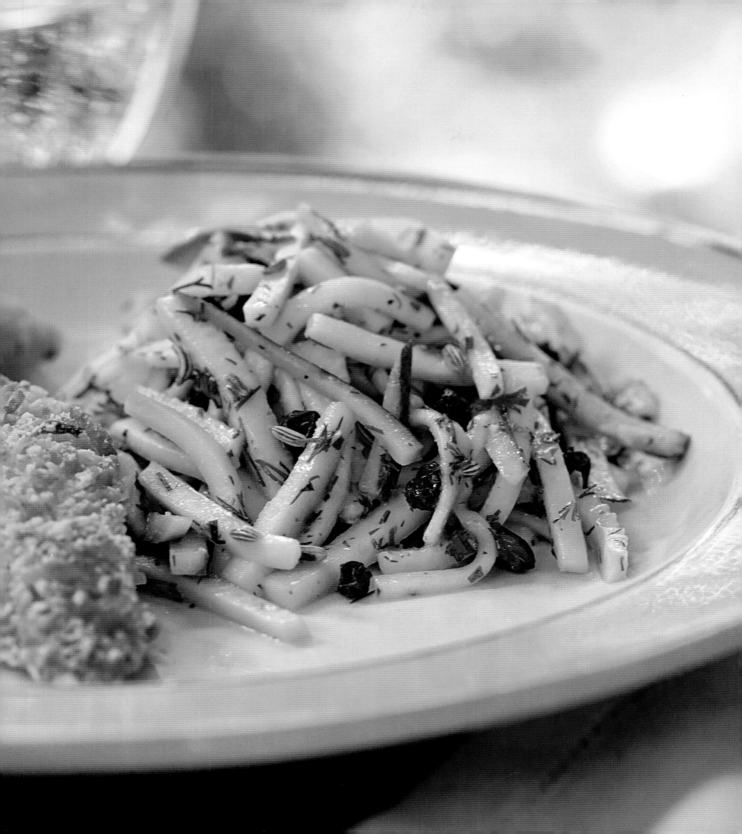

# BEST-BY-THE-BATCH CARAMELIZED ONIONS

Caramelized onions possess an unparalleled flavor that can be achieved only with ample prep. When you have time, make a double and triple batch to freeze so you can always have this tasty accompaniment on hand as a side for meats, topping for pizza, added to a sandwich, or tossed with pasta.

**¾ cup (175 ml) balsamic vinegar**

**⅔ cup (160 ml) olive oil**

**2 tablespoons (26 g) granulated sugar**

**12 small mild onions, peeled, trimmed**

① Preheat oven to 425°F (220°C, or gas mark 7). Grease a 9 x 11-inch (23 x 28 cm) baking dish.

② In a small bowl, whisk together vinegar, oil, and sugar. Place onions in the baking dish and drizzle with vinegar mixture. Stir to coat well. Cover baking dish with aluminum foil. Bake for 40 minutes.

③ Remove foil and move dish to the bottom rack. Bake for 30 more minutes or until sauce is thickened in the bottom of the dish. Roll onions in sauce. Let cool and then refrigerate until cold.

YIELD: 12 SERVINGS

 ## TO FREEZE

INDIVIDUAL SERVINGS: Place each onion, drizzled with sauce, in a freezer- and microwave-safe container.

FOR A CROWD: Transfer onions and sauce to two 1-gallon (3.8 L) freezer bags, removing as much air as possible before sealing.

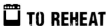 ## TO REHEAT

Thaw onions overnight in the refrigerator.

MICROWAVE METHOD: Reheat individual servings on high for 2 minutes or until heated through.

OVEN METHOD: Preheat oven to 350°F (180°C, or gas mark 4). Place onions and sauce in original baking dish and bake for 20 minutes or until heated through.

## NUTRITION SPOTLIGHT: AWESOME ONIONS

Onions provide more than 20% of the Daily Value of chromium, a mineral that helps cells respond to insulin, which can help balance blood sugar levels and is associated with heart health. Onions are also rich in sulfur-containing compounds and flavanoids, which are linked with fighting cancer and reducing inflammation. They may even reduce the carcinogens in meats that are produced from high-heat cooking; instead of stir-frying meat alone, stir-fry it with sliced onions.

AMOUNT PER SERVING: Calories 156.29; Total Fat 12.08 g; Cholesterol 0 mg; Sodium 6.71 mg; Potassium 120.21 mg; Total Carbohydrates 11.35 g; Fiber 1.19 g; Sugar 7.45 g; Protein 0.85 g

# TENDER ROASTED VEGETABLES * *Try*

Roasting vegetables is one of the best ways to bring out the wonderfully varied flavors of vegetables, giving them a caramelized deliciousness that makes them irresistible at the table. For an eco-friendly nutritional boost, eat with the seasons and roast only the vegetables that are in season in your area. Roasted root vegetables in the fall and winter are especially delish!

1 pound (455 g) zucchini, diced

1 pound (455 g) yellow squash, diced

1 red onion, halved, sliced

1 red bell pepper, seeded, sliced

2 bunches radishes, trimmed, halved

3 tablespoons (45 ml) olive oil

Salt and freshly ground black pepper to taste

① Preheat oven to 450°F (230°C, or gas mark 8). In a large bowl, toss together vegetables and oil to coat. Season with salt and pepper. Spread vegetables in a single layer in a jelly-roll pan.

② Roast for 20 minutes, stir with a spatula, and roast 15 to 20 minutes more or until vegetables are lightly browned and tender. Let vegetables cool completely.

YIELD: 12 CUPS (2.2 KG), OR 12 SERVINGS

## COOKING TIP: EAT WITH THE SEASONS

Eating locally and with the seasons not only supports your local farmers and economy, it is also healthier for your family and kind to the environment. When you buy out-of-season produce, it is likely transported from far away, meaning it won't have as many nutrients or be as fresh as locally picked produce and it also creates a large carbon footprint. Frequent your local farmers' market, join a CSA, and feed your family local, seasonal produce.

 ## TO FREEZE

INDIVIDUAL SERVINGS: Transfer vegetables to single-serving airtight containers or 1-quart (950 ml) freezer bags.

FOR A CROWD: Transfer vegetables to 1-gallon (3.8 L)freezer bags.

 ## TO REHEAT

Let vegetables thaw in the refrigerator overnight.

MICROWAVE METHOD: Reheat single-serving portions of vegetables in the microwave on high for 2 to 3 minutes. Drain off extra liquid. Reheat large portions of vegetables on high for 5 minutes. Drain off extra liquid.

STOVETOP METHOD: Place vegetables in a skillet over medium heat and cook, stirring often, for 7 to 9 minutes or until vegetables are heated through and excess liquid evaporates.

AMOUNT PER SERVING: Calories 60; Total Fat 3.54 g; Cholesterol 0 mg; Sodium 13.16 mg; Potassium 296.45 mg; Total Carbohydrates 7.21 g; Fiber 1.66 g; Sugar 1.3 g; Protein 1.1 g

# FAST AND FABULOUS FAVA BEANS

High in fiber and folic acid, fava beans—also called broad beans—are one of summer's most coveted treats. In season for only a couple of months, fava beans can be snatched up at farmers' markets and then kept in your freezer for enjoyment year-round. This side dish joins tender favas with other flavorful vegetables and white wine that pairs wonderfully with rice, pasta, meat, and poultry dishes.

2 tablespoons (28 ml) olive oil

1 medium onion, finely chopped

1 clove garlic, thinly sliced

2 pounds (900 g) shelled fava beans

1 cup (110 g) sun-dried tomatoes packed in olive oil, drained, chopped

2 carrots, sliced

⅓ cup (80 ml) dry white wine

2 tablespoons (8 g) chopped fresh parsley

1 bay leaf

Salt and freshly ground black pepper to taste

① Heat oil in a Dutch oven over medium heat. Add onion and cook, stirring often, for 5 minutes. Add garlic and cook, stirring, for 30 seconds.

② Add fava beans, sun-dried tomatoes, and carrots, stirring to combine. Cook, stirring occasionally, until carrots are just tender.

③ Add wine, parsley, and bay leaf. Cook, stirring occasionally, for 3 minutes. Season with salt and pepper. Reduce heat to low and cook for 5 more minutes. Remove the bay leaf. Cool completely.

YIELD: 10 CUPS (1 KG), OR 8 SERVINGS

## COOKING TIP: FREEZE FRESH FAVAS

Freeze fava beans so you have a ready supply in your freezer: Put a large pot of salted water over high heat to boil. Rinse fava beans well, removing any debris. Shell the beans, sliding fava beans out of the pod and into a bowl. Pour fava beans into boiling water and boil for 3 minutes. Drain and immediately plunge fava beans into a bowl of ice water to halt cooking. Drain in a colander again. Transfer beans to a stack of paper towels or a dish towel. Use your fingernails to remove skins from beans. Place cooled favas on a rimmed baking sheet and freeze until solid. Transfer to a large freezer bag.

##  TO FREEZE

INDIVIDUAL SERVINGS: Divide fava beans into eight 1-quart (950 ml) freezer bags or freezer- and microwave-safe containers and freeze.

FOR A CROWD: Place fava beans in a 1-gallon (3.8 L) freezer bag, removing as much air as possible before sealing. Lay bag flat in a casserole dish and freeze. When solid, remove casserole dish.

##  TO REHEAT

Thaw fava beans in refrigerator overnight.

MICROWAVE METHOD: Reheat individual portions in the microwave on high for 1 to 2 minutes or until heated through.

STOVETOP METHOD: Reheat beans in a Dutch oven over medium-high heat, stirring often, until heated through.

AMOUNT PER SERVING: Calories 469.7; Total Fat 6.6 g; Cholesterol 0 mg; Sodium 66.84 mg; Potassium 1523.95 mg; Total Carbohydrates 73.58 g; Fiber 30.71 g; Sugar 7.76 g; Protein 31.37 g

# EASY CHEESY HERBED POLENTA ✳

Polenta is essentially coarsely ground corn simply simmered in liquid until it becomes a creamy side for roasted meats, poultry, and seafood as well as hearty stews and sautéed vegetables. Polenta has an affinity for rich tomato sauces and can become a quick main meal when topped with Must-Make Marinara Sauce (page 166) and sprinkled with cheese.

3 tablespoons (45 ml) olive oil

2 cups (320 g) finely chopped red onion

½ teaspoon salt

Freshly ground black pepper to taste

3 cloves garlic, minced

8 cups (1.9 L) water

2 cups (275 g) coarse ground cornmeal

6 tablespoons (85 g) unsalted butter

2 cups (200 g) grated Parmesan cheese

2 tablespoons (8 g) finely chopped fresh oregano

2 tablespoons (8 g) finely chopped fresh parsley

2 tablespoons (8 g) finely chopped fresh tarragon

① Heat oil in a large saucepan over medium heat. Add onion and cook, stirring often, for 4 minutes. Season with salt and pepper and stir in garlic. Cook, stirring constantly, for 30 seconds.

② Turn the heat up to high and add water. Gradually add cornmeal, whisking constantly. Bring to a boil and then reduce heat to medium-low and continue to whisk until mixture starts to thicken.

③ Whisk in butter and cheese. Continue to cook, whisking constantly, until butter and cheese is melted. Whisk in herbs and remove from heat. Season with salt and pepper. Cool completely.

YIELD: 8 TO 10 SERVINGS

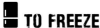 ## TO FREEZE

INDIVIDUAL SERVINGS: Divide mixture into 8 to 10 freezer- and microwave-safe containers. Let cool completely before sealing and freezing.

FOR A CROWD: Line a 13 x 9-inch (33 x 23 cm) baking dish with enough freezer wrap to generously cover the bottom, sides, and overlap the top. Pour warm polenta into dish, spreading it out evenly. Let cool completely. Fold freezer wrap over and seal the edges. Freeze until solid and then remove baking dish.

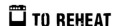 ## TO REHEAT

Let individual servings of polenta thaw in refrigerator overnight. Before thawing large portion, remove freezer wrap, place frozen polenta in original baking dish, and then thaw in refrigerator.

MICROWAVE METHOD: Individual servings can be reheated in the microwave on high for 1 to 2 minutes or until heated through.

OVEN METHOD: Preheat oven to 350°F (180°C, or gas mark 4). Cover baking dish with foil and bake for 15 to 20 minutes or until heated through. Cut polenta into squares to serve.

STOVETOP METHOD: For a creamier polenta, place thawed polenta into a saucepan over medium heat. Add ¼ to ½ cup (60 to 120 ml) water or broth, stirring and adding more liquid until you reach desired consistency.

### SERVING SUGGESTIONS

- Top your polenta with sautéed garlic and greens and sprinkle with goat cheese.
- Add braised leeks and fennel and sprinkle with toasted walnuts or pecans.
- Stir in Five-Ways Fresh Herb Spread (page 170), Toasted Almond and Basil Pesto (page 169), or Hazelnut and Sun-Dried Tomato Pesto (page 167).
- Stir in mascarpone cheese and cooked sausage.
- For a sweet polenta, simmer water and cornmeal until creamy and then swirl in berries, half-and-half, and honey.

AMOUNT PER SERVING: Calories 284.89; Total Fat 17.63 g; Cholesterol 35.92 mg; Sodium 449.46 mg; Potassium 111.34 mg; Total Carbohydrates 22.53 g; Fiber 2.46 g; Sugar 0.36 g; Protein 10.2 g

# SMASHED GARLIC POTATOES

Though raw potatoes don't freeze well, mashed potatoes are a convenient side to keep on hand in the freezer, whether you want a single serving or need to feed a crowd. Adding garlic and garlic chives gives them an extra dimension of flavor that elevates them above plain mashed spuds.

**3½ pounds (1.6 kg) Yukon gold potatoes, peeled, quartered**

**½ cup (115 g) Neufchâtel cheese**

**¾ cup (173 g) sour cream**

**1 teaspoon salt**

**Freshly ground black pepper to taste**

**3 cloves garlic, pressed**

**4 tablespoons (55 g) unsalted butter, sliced**

**2 tablespoons (6 g) or more minced fresh garlic chives**

① Place potatoes in a large pot of salted cold water and bring to a boil over high heat. Cook for 30 minutes or until potatoes are tender. Drain and return potatoes to the pot.

② Using a masher, start to break up the potatoes. Add cheese, sour cream, salt, pepper, garlic, and butter, using an electric mixer on low speed to blend. Increase speed as ingredients come together. Stir in chives. Continue to blend until smooth. Let cool completely.

YIELD: 8 CUPS (1.8 KG), OR 16 SERVINGS

## SERVING SUGGESTIONS

Here are a few things you can do with your mashed potatoes:

- Spread on top of a shepherd's pie.
- Whisk with eggs and a little milk for potato pancakes.
- Use as a thickener or the base for a creamy soup.
- Mix with bread crumbs and cheese, form into balls, spray with oil, and bake.
- Make twice-baked potatoes by mixing mashed potatoes with herbs, cooked crumbled sausage, and cheese and baking until lightly browned.

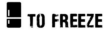 **TO FREEZE**

INDIVIDUAL SERVINGS: Divide potatoes into freezer- and microwave-safe containers.

FOR A CROWD: Place potatoes in a 9 x 11-inch (23 x 28 cm) baking dish. Place in the freezer until firm. Place a sheet of plastic wrap directly on potatoes. Tightly wrap baking dish with foil.

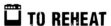 **TO REHEAT**

Let potatoes thaw in the refrigerator overnight.

MICROWAVE METHOD: Reheat individual servings in the microwave on high for 1 to 2 minutes or until heated through.

OVEN METHOD: Preheat oven to 350°F (180°C, or gas mark 4). Remove foil and plastic from baking dish and bake in the oven for 30 minutes or until heated through.

AMOUNT PER SERVING: Calories 134.47; Total Fat 6.74 g; Cholesterol 17.61 mg; Sodium 180.24 mg; Potassium 510.7 mg; Total Carbohydrates 18.31 g; Fiber 2.03 g; Sugar 2.04 g; Protein 3.82 g

# OVEN-BAKED HUSH PUPPIES

Though traditionally deep fried, this healthier version of hush puppies is not only baked, it utilizes a muffin pan, which lends itself to easier mess-free batch cooking. Hush puppies are typically served with a seafood dinner, offering an alternative to plain bread or other starchy foods, such as rice.

¼ cup (60 ml) vegetable oil

1¾ cups (245 g) cornmeal

½ cup (60 g) white whole-wheat flour

¼ cup (31 g) all-purpose flour

1 tablespoon (14 g) baking powder

1 teaspoon baking soda

1 teaspoon salt

Pinch of cayenne pepper

1 egg

1½ cups (355 ml) buttermilk

⅓ cup (20 g) finely chopped fresh parsley

① Preheat oven to 425°F (220°C, or gas mark 7). Drizzle a little oil in the bottom of each cup in a 12-cup muffin pan. Turn pan to coat sides of cups. Place muffin pan in oven to heat.

② In a large bowl, whisk together cornmeal, flour, baking powder, baking soda, salt, and cayenne. Set aside.

③ In a medium bowl, lightly beat egg. Whisk in buttermilk and parsley. Add buttermilk mixture to cornmeal mixture. Stir until just moistened.

④ Remove muffin pan from oven and spoon batter into muffin cups. Bake for 12 minutes or until hush puppies are just cooked through.

YIELD: 12 HUSH PUPPIES, OR 12 SERVINGS

 **TO FREEZE**

Remove hush puppies from pan and let cool completely on a wire rack. Place on a baking sheet and freeze. Transfer to a 1-gallon (3.8 L) freezer bag and seal, removing as much air as possible.

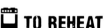 **TO REHEAT**

Let thaw in the refrigerator.

OVEN METHOD: Preheat oven to 350°F (180°C, or gas mark 4). Place hush puppies on a baking sheet and bake for 5 to 8 minutes or until heated through.

AMOUNT PER SERVING: Calories 373.18; Total Fat 6.64 g; Cholesterol 18.64 mg; Sodium 464.31 mg; Potassium 183.2 mg; Total Carbohydrates 67.94 g; Fiber 3.34 g; Sugar 1.58 g; Protein 9.92 g

# FAMILY-FAVORITE FREEZER RICE

Refined 5-minute rice from a box offers little nutritional value, yet steaming brown, wild, and other unprocessed varieties of rice can take up to almost an hour. The most convenient way to serve wholesome types of rice with your family's meals is by cooking large batches in advance and keeping them in your freezer.

**2 cups (380 g) brown rice**

**4 cups (950 ml) water or broth**

① Bring rice and water or broth to a boil over medium-high heat. Reduce heat to low, cover, and cook for 45 to 50 minutes or until water is just absorbed. Do not overcook. Spread rice out on a baking sheet and let cool completely.

YIELD: 4 CUPS (660 G), OR 8 SERVINGS

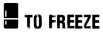 TO FREEZE

INDIVIDUAL SERVINGS: Freeze rice on the baking sheet until solid and divide among 8 freezer- and microwave-safe containers or 1-quart (950 ml) freezer bags.

FOR A CROWD: Freeze rice on the baking sheet until solid and then transfer to a large freezer bag, removing as much air as possible before sealing.

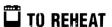 TO REHEAT

Let rice thaw in refrigerator overnight.

MICROWAVE METHOD: For individual servings, add a little water to rice. Reheat on high, stirring every minute, for 2 to 3 minutes or until heated through.

STOVETOP METHOD: Place rice in a saucepan over medium heat and add enough water to just moisten rice. Cook, stirring often, until heated through.

AMOUNT PER SERVING: Calories 58.33; Total Fat 1.04 g; Cholesterol 0 mg; Sodium 383.39 mg; Potassium 103.2 mg; Total Carbohydrates 8.53 g; Fiber 0.72 g; Sugar 0.53 g; Protein 3.32 g

# GINGER AND VEGGIE FRIED RICE

Fried rice is a tasty side for Asian meals, but this rendition, showcasing protein-rich eggs and edamame, can also be eaten as a main meal if you want a one-dish dinner.

**3 tablespoons (45 ml) olive oil, divided**

**6 eggs, well-beaten**

**6 tablespoons (48 g) sesame seeds**

**3 thin slices peeled fresh ginger, finely chopped**

**1 cup (160 g) thinly sliced onion**

**1 cup (120 g) thinly sliced celery**

**1 bunch shredded spinach leaves**

**1 cup (150 g) edamame**

**4 to 5 cups (780 to 995 g) cooked brown rice**

**Tamari sauce to taste**

① Heat 1 tablespoon (15 ml) oil in a large nonstick skillet over medium heat. Pour eggs into skillet and swirl to evenly coat bottom of skillet. Cover skillet and cook for 1 to 2 minutes or until eggs are just cooked through. Coarsely chop eggs and set aside.

② Add remaining oil to a Dutch oven and set over medium heat. Scatter sesame seeds and ginger into pan and cook, stirring, for 1 minute. Add onions and celery and cook, stirring often, for 5 minutes.

③ Stir in spinach leaves and edamame. Cook, stirring occasionally, until spinach is wilted. Stir in rice and cook until heated through.

④ Add eggs and tamari, stirring to combine. Remove from heat and spread fried rice in a rimmed baking sheet. Cool completely.

YIELD: 8 TO 9 CUPS (1.3 TO 1.5 KG), OR 8 SERVINGS

## COOKING TIP: FREEZE WHOLE GRAINS

Rice isn't the only grain you can fix and freeze. You can also make large batches of quinoa, barley, bulgur, millet, as well as any shape whole-wheat pasta. Simply cook grains for 1 to 2 minutes less than package directions, spread flat on a baking sheet, and freeze until firm. Transfer to freezer bags or freezer containers in portions of your choice. To cook, thaw grain or product in refrigerator overnight and reheat.

## TO FREEZE

INDIVIDUAL SERVINGS: Divide rice into freezer- and microwave-safe containers and place in the freezer.

FOR A CROWD: Place rice in a 1-gallon (3.8 L) freezer bag, lay bag flat in a casserole dish, and freeze. When solid, remove casserole dish.

## TO REHEAT

Thaw rice in refrigerator overnight.

MICROWAVE METHOD: Reheat individual servings of rice in the microwave on high for 2 minutes or until rice is heated through.

OVEN METHOD: Preheat oven to 350°F (180°C, or gas mark 4). Transfer rice to a 9 x 13-inch (23 x 33 cm) baking dish and cover with foil. Bake for 15 minutes or until heated through.

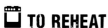

AMOUNT PER SERVING: Calories 266.45; Total Fat 13.72 g; Cholesterol 158.63 mg; Sodium 105.1 mg; Potassium 477.53 mg; Total Carbohydrates 26.35 g; Fiber 4.83 g; Sugar 2.51 g; Protein 11.37 g

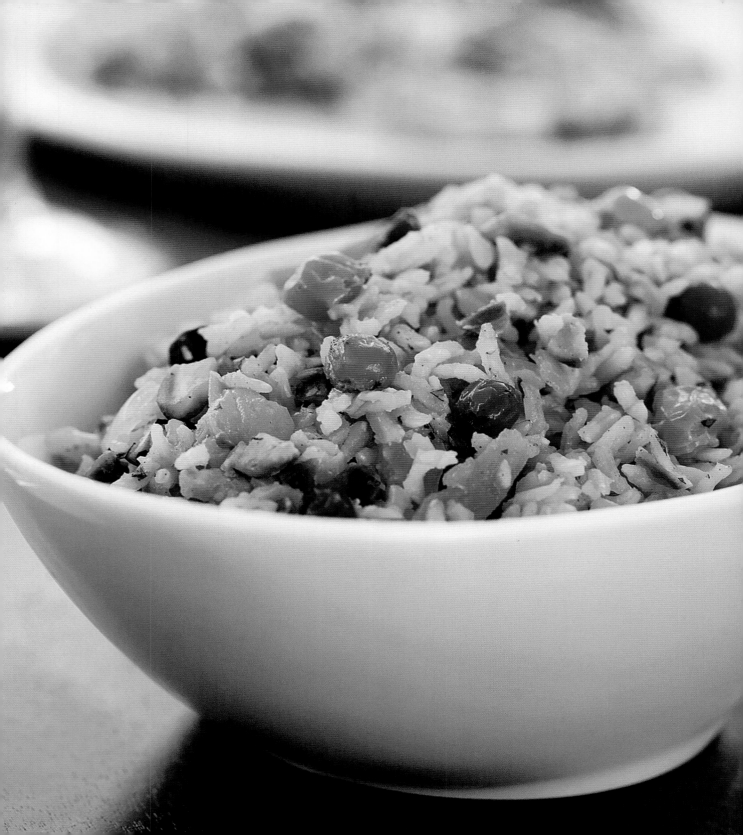

# APRICOT-PISTACHIO RICE PILAF

Apricots and pistachios give this pilaf a nutritional lift while providing nutty crunch and dried fruit chew. Though pilafs are typically loaded with butter fat, this one keeps butter to a bare minimum and punches up the flavor with spices, herbs, dried fruit, and nuts.

**1 tablespoon (14 g) unsalted butter**

**1 tablespoon (15 ml) olive oil**

**1 medium onion, chopped**

**1½ cups (285 g) brown basmati rice**

**½ teaspoon ground cardamom**

**2 teaspoons minced fresh rosemary**

**Salt and freshly ground black pepper to taste**

**3½ cups (820 ml) reduced-sodium vegetable broth**

**½ cup (75 g) golden raisins**

**⅓ cup (43 g) sliced dried apricot halves**

**1¼ cups (185 g) shelled pistachios, chopped**

**½ cup (30 g) finely chopped fresh parsley**

 Heat butter and olive oil in a large saucepan over medium heat, swirling pan until butter is melted. Add onion, rice, cardamom, and rosemary and cook, stirring often, until onion is softened and rice is toasted, about 7 minutes. Season with salt and pepper.

 Stir in broth, raisins, and apricots and bring to a boil. Reduce heat to medium-low. Cover and simmer until broth is absorbed, about 25 minutes. Remove from heat and let stand 5 minutes. Stir in pistachios and parsley. Spread out on a rimmed baking sheet and let cool completely.

YIELD: 8 SERVINGS

## NUTRITION SPOTLIGHT: PISTACHIOS

Known to improve heart health by reducing inflammation and cholesterol, pistachios are also a quality source of protein, fiber, good-for-you fat, and an array of vitamins and minerals. Research suggests that eating 1.5 ounces (43 g) of nuts, like pistachios, a day can reduce the risk of heart disease. Add pistachios to desserts, grain dishes, baked goods, salads, vegetables, and sauces or use nuts to crust fish and poultry.

## TO FREEZE

INDIVIDUAL SERVINGS: Divide pilaf among 8 freezer- and microwave-safe containers or 1-quart (950 ml) freezer bags.

FOR A CROWD: Place rice in a large freezer bag, removing as much air as possible before sealing.

## TO REHEAT

Let rice thaw in refrigerator overnight.

MICROWAVE METHOD: Reheat individual servings of rice in the microwave on high for 2 minutes or until heated through.

OVEN METHOD: Preheat oven to 350°F (180°C, or gas mark 4). Pour rice in a baking dish and cover with foil. Bake for 20 minutes or until heated through.

AMOUNT PER SERVING: Calories 345.68; Total Fat 11.71 g; Cholesterol 3.82 mg; Sodium 498.14 mg; Potassium 322.61 mg; Total Carbohydrates 43.01 g; Fiber 4.41 g; Sugar 11.14 g; Protein 6.59 g

# FIX-AND-FREEZE HERB STUFFING

Stuffing isn't just for special occasions and holidays. By keeping a ready supply in your freezer, you can have yummy sides of stuffing for your everyday chicken or meat dishes. Healthier than stuffing out of a box, this herbalicious recipe can be on the table in 30 minutes or less.

3 tablespoons (45 ml) canola oil

2 onions, finely chopped

2 stalks celery, finely chopped

2 carrots, finely chopped

2 cloves garlic, minced

3 tablespoons (6 g) dried sage, crumbled

1 tablespoon (3 g) dried rosemary

1 tablespoon (3 g) dried thyme

1 teaspoon salt

Freshly ground black pepper to taste

1 large loaf day-old French or sourdough bread, cubed

4 cups (950 ml) low-sodium vegetable or chicken broth

① In a Dutch oven, heat oil over medium-high heat. Add onions, celery, and carrots and cook, stirring often, until vegetables are softened and turning golden. Add garlic, sage, rosemary, thyme, salt, and pepper and cook, stirring, for 1 minute.

② Add bread and toss to coat. Pour in broth, tossing to coat, adding more or less, to moisten. Stuffing should not be soggy.

YIELD: 16 CUPS, OR 20 SERVINGS

## COOKING TIP: FREEZE FRESH HERBS

Your extra bounty of herbs can be quickly preserved by freezing. Though they won't retain the crispness of fresh-picked herbs, their lovely flavor will remain intact. Here's how to freeze fresh herbs: Rinse herbs and pat dry with paper towels. Spread herbs in one layer on a baking sheet, cover with plastic wrap, and freeze until solid. Transfer frozen herbs to freezer bags, removing as much air as possible before sealing.

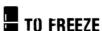 TO FREEZE

INDIVIDUAL SERVINGS: Divide stuffing among 10 to 20 freezer- and microwave-safe containers.

FOR A CROWD: Place stuffing in 1-gallon (3.8 L) freezer bags and lay flat in a casserole dish. Freeze until solid, then remove casserole dish.

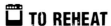 TO REHEAT

Let stuffing thaw for a few hours in the refrigerator.

MICROWAVE METHOD: Reheat stuffing in the microwave on high for 1 to 2 minutes or until heated through.

OVEN METHOD: Preheat oven to 375°F (190°C, or gas mark 5). Transfer stuffing to a baking dish, cover with foil, and bake for 20 minutes. Remove foil and bake for 10 more minutes or until top is lightly browned, if desired.

AMOUNT PER SERVING: Calories 123.32; Total Fat 2.6 g; Cholesterol 0 mg; Sodium 499.27 mg; Potassium 91.57 mg; Total Carbohydrates 15.32 g; Fiber 1.3 g; Sugar 1.58 g; Protein 2.98 g

*? TM*

# ITALIAN MEAT(LESS)BALLS

Adopting a vegetarian diet doesn't mean nixing meatballs from your diet. It simply requires a creative, grain- and vegetable-based change in ingredients. This recipe gives you a high-fiber alternative that is equally delicious paired with a flavorful marinara sauce. Garnish with freshly grated Parmesan cheese and you've got the perfect meat-free Italian meal.

**4 cups (780 g) cooked long-grain brown rice**

**1 cup (80 g) quick-cooking oats, ground**

**1 medium red onion, finely chopped**

**4 cloves garlic, minced**

**⅔ cup (77 g) dry whole-wheat bread crumbs**

**4 eggs, beaten**

**⅔ cup (160 ml) milk**

**¼ cup (28 g) ground flaxseed**

**2 tablespoons (12 g) Italian seasoning**

**Salt to taste**

**½ teaspoon freshly ground black pepper**

**¼ teaspoon cayenne pepper**

**½ cup (58 g) wheat germ**

**2 to 3 tablespoons (28 to 45 ml) canola oil**

**2 jars (28 ounces, or 785 g, each) tomato sauce**

① In a large bowl, mix together rice, oats, onion, garlic, bread crumbs, eggs, milk, ground flax, Italian seasoning, salt, pepper, and cayenne.

② Cover bowl and refrigerate for at least 1 hour. Shape mixture into 50 meatballs and roll each in wheat germ to coat.

③ Heat 2 tablespoons (28 ml) oil in a large nonstick skillet over medium heat. In 2 batches, cook meatballs for 8 to 10 minutes, turning occasionally, until light golden brown, adding more oil if needed.

④ Drain meatballs on paper towels and allow to cool completely. Gently mix meatballs with tomato sauce.

YIELD: 10 SERVINGS

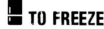 **TO FREEZE**

INDIVIDUAL SERVINGS: Divide meatballs and sauce into ten 1-quart (950 ml) freezer bags or freezer- and microwave-safe containers (about 5 meatballs and ½ cup [123 g] sauce), removing as much air as possible before sealing.

FOR A CROWD: Place mixture in a 1-gallon (3.8 L) freezer bag, lay bag flat in a casserole dish and place in the freezer. When mixture is frozen, remove casserole dish.

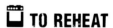 **TO REHEAT**

Thaw meatballs overnight in refrigerator.

MICROWAVE METHOD: Reheat individual servings in the microwave on high for 3 minutes or until heated through.

STOVETOP METHOD: Reheat individual servings or entire recipe in a saucepan over medium-low heat, stirring occasionally, until meatballs are heated through.

AMOUNT PER SERVING: Calories 282.63; Total Fat 9.8 g; Cholesterol 85.9 mg; Sodium 871.23 mg; Potassium 682.1 mg; Total Carbohydrates 40.46 g; Fiber 6.99 g; Sugar 8.44 g; Protein 11.09 g

# ANYTIME CABBAGE AND APPLE TURNOVERS

Plump with tender shredded cabbage and apples, these savory turnovers are a satisfying lunch or meat-free main course meal.

FOR THE PASTRY:

**8 ounces (225 g) Neufchâtel, softened at room temperature**

**½ cup (112 g) unsalted butter, softened at room temperature**

**1½ cups (180 g) whole-wheat pastry flour**

FOR THE VEGETABLE FILLING:

**2 tablespoons (28 ml) canola oil**

**1 onion, finely chopped**

**2 cloves garlic, minced**

**4 cups (280 g) finely shredded red cabbage**

**2 Granny Smith apples, cored, finely grated**

**Juice of 1 lemon**

**1 tablespoon (20 g) honey**

**⅓ cup (33 g) toasted walnuts or pecans, chopped**

**2 tablespoons (28 ml) apple cider vinegar**

**1 teaspoon prepared horseradish**

**Salt and freshly ground black pepper to taste**

① For the pastry, in a standup mixer fitted with the paddle attachment, beat Neufchâtel and butter until smooth. Add flour and blend until a dough forms. Scrape dough onto a lightly floured surface and form into a disk. Wrap with plastic and refrigerate for 30 minutes.

② Preheat oven to 350°F (180°C, or gas mark 4).

③ For the filling, heat oil in a large skillet over medium-high heat. Add onion and cook, stirring, for 2 minutes. Add garlic and cook, stirring, for 1 minute. Add cabbage and cook, stirring occasionally, for 5 to 6 minutes or until cabbage is tender. Add apple and lemon juice and cook, stirring, for 1 minute.

④ Add walnuts, vinegar, and horseradish, stirring for 2 minutes. Season with salt and pepper. Remove from heat.

⑤ On a lightly floured surface or between 2 pieces of plastic wrap, roll dough out and using a 3- to 4-inch (7.5 to 10 cm) biscuit cutter, cut into 36 circles. Place filling on half of each circle and fold the other half of the dough over the filling. Use the back of a fork to seal edges.

⑥ Poke holes in the top of each turnover. Bake for 15 minutes. Remove from the oven and let cool completely on a wire rack.

YIELD: 36 TURNOVERS, OR 12 SERVINGS

## COOKING TIP: FREEZING CABBAGE

Stock up on fresh cabbage and keep it in your freezer. Here's how to freeze cabbage: Shred cabbage with the food processor blade or thinly slice it with a knife. Blanch in boiling water for 2 minutes, drain, and then spread out on paper towels to dry. Pat dry with additional paper towels. When fully dry, spread out on a rimmed baking sheet and freeze. Store in freezer bags. You can thaw cabbage or add frozen cabbage directly to recipes.

AMOUNT PER SERVING: Calories 239.7; Total Fat 16.54 g; Cholesterol 34.44 mg; Sodium 83.8 mg; Potassium 191.79 mg; Total Carbohydrates 20.8 g; Fiber 4.11 g; Sugar 4.83 g; Protein 5.12 g

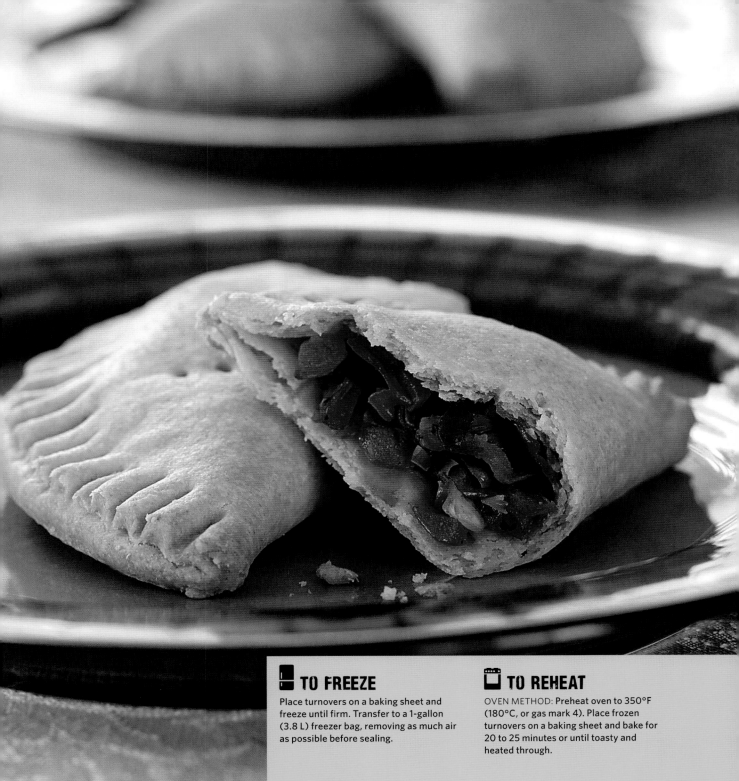

## TO FREEZE

Place turnovers on a baking sheet and freeze until firm. Transfer to a 1-gallon (3.8 L) freezer bag, removing as much air as possible before sealing.

## TO REHEAT

OVEN METHOD: Preheat oven to 350°F (180°C, or gas mark 4). Place frozen turnovers on a baking sheet and bake for 20 to 25 minutes or until toasty and heated through.

# WEEKNIGHT STUFFED SHELLS

Jumbo pasta shells stuffed with three cheeses, vegetables, and herbs is a hearty vegetarian main meal that can be on the table in less than the time it would take you to call for a vegetarian takeout pizza.

24 uncooked jumbo pasta shells

1 can (10 ounces, or 280 g) vegetable broth

1 carrot, shredded

1 bunch radishes, diced

1 small onion, finely chopped

2 cups (500 g) part-skim ricotta cheese

½ cup (60 g) shredded mozzarella cheese

1 egg

½ cup (50 g) freshly grated Parmesan cheese

1 teaspoon dried oregano

1 teaspoon dried basil

3 tablespoons (12 g) finely chopped fresh parsley

1 jar (28 ounces, or 785 g) spaghetti sauce

① Cook shells until just al dente, about 11 minutes. Rinse, drain, and let cool.

② In a large saucepan over medium-high heat, bring broth to a boil. Stir in carrots, radishes, and onions and cook 3 to 4 minutes or until vegetables are tender.

③ Drain vegetables in a colander and transfer to a large bowl. Add ricotta, mozzarella, egg, and Parmesan cheese in a large bowl. Stir in herbs.

④ Fill each pasta shell with vegetable mixture. The vegetable mixture may still be warm, so let stuffed shells cool completely. You won't cook shells and sauce until you reheat after freezing.

YIELD: 8 SERVINGS

## BONUS RECIPE: CHICKPEA ARTICHOKE SALAD

- 1 can (15 ounces, or 425 g) chickpeas or garbanzo beans, rinsed, drained
- 1 cup (300 g) marinated artichoke hearts, drained, coarsely chopped
- ½ cup (55 g) sun-dried tomatoes packed in olive oil, coarsely chopped
- 3 tablespoons (12 g) finely chopped fresh parsley
- Salt and freshly ground black pepper
- Shaved Parmesan to taste
- Large whole radicchio leaves

In a large bowl, toss chickpeas, artichoke hearts, tomatoes, parsley, and salt and pepper until well-combined. Add Parmesan and toss again. Place a radicchio leaf on each plate and fill with salad.

## TO FREEZE

INDIVIDUAL SERVINGS: Divide shells (3 per serving) among eight 1-quart (950 ml) freezer bags or freezer- and microwave-safe containers. Pour about ½ cup (123 g) tomato sauce over shells. Remove as much air as possible and seal bag or container.

FOR A CROWD: Line a 9 x 13-inch (23 x 33 cm) baking dish with freezer paper large enough to cover bottom, overlap the sides, and extend over the top of dish. Pour about 1 cup (245 g) tomato sauce in dish, spreading it around to evenly coat. Arrange stuffed shells in sauce and cover with remaining sauce. Loosely cover and place in the freezer until solid. Lift freezer paper out of dish and tightly seal the top and sides. Place back in the freezer.

## TO REHEAT

Place individual servings of shells in the refrigerator to thaw. For larger servings, unwrap frozen shells and sauce and place in a 9 x 13-inch (23 x 33 cm) casserole dish to thaw in the refrigerator overnight.

MICROWAVE METHOD: Reheat individual servings of shells in the microwave on high for 2 to 3 minutes or until heated through.

OVEN METHOD: Preheat oven to 350°F (180°C, or gas mark 4). Cover dish with foil. Bake for 30 minutes. Remove foil and bake 10 minutes or until hot and bubbly.

Serve with shredded mozzarella or Parmesan on top.

AMOUNT PER SERVING: Calories 372.98; Total Fat 12.46 g; Cholesterol 58.45 mg; Sodium 883.68 mg; Potassium 575.6 mg; Total Carbohydrates 46.87 g; Fiber 5.21 g; Sugar 10.57 g; Protein 18.8 g

# CHEESY GRITS WITH SAUTÉED ONIONS AND MUSHROOMS

Creamy cheesy grits topped with naturally sweet caramelized onions and earthy-flavored wild mushrooms is one of my favorite vegetarian meals. Every satisfying bite warms both my belly and soul. When I want comfort for my carnivoristic cravings, I simply add cooked duck, roasted chicken, or turkey sausage.

FOR THE GRITS:

**2 cups (275 g) medium-grain yellow cornmeal**

**7 cups (1.6 L) water**

**Salt and freshly ground black pepper**

**1 teaspoon dried oregano**

**¼ cup (55 g) unsalted butter**

**1 cup (80 g) shaved Parmesan**

**1 cup (110 g) shredded fontina cheese**

**3 tablespoons (12 g) finely chopped fresh parsley**

FOR THE SAUTÉED ONIONS AND MUSHROOMS:

**2 tablespoons (28 ml) olive oil**

**2 onions, halved, very thinly sliced**

**1½ pounds (680 g) sliced wild mushrooms such as shiitake, porcini, chanterelles, or morels**

**Salt and freshly ground black pepper**

**1 cup (110 g) chopped sun-dried tomatoes packed in olive oil**

① In a large pot over high heat, whisk together cornmeal and water. Bring to a boil, whisking constantly, and reduce heat to medium-low. Cook, whisking constantly, until cornmeal thickens. Stir in salt and pepper and oregano. Remove from heat and whisk in butter, cheeses, and parsley. Set aside to cool completely.

② Heat oil in a large skillet over medium-high heat. Add onion and mushrooms and season with salt and pepper. Cook, stirring occasionally, for 5 minutes. Add tomatoes and cook, stirring occasionally, for 5 to 6 more minutes. Set aside to cool completely.

YIELD: 8 SERVINGS

## 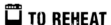 TO FREEZE

INDIVIDUAL SERVINGS: Divide grits into 8 freezer- and microwave-safe containers. Top with onion and mushroom mixture. Seal and freeze.

FOR A CROWD: Line a 13 x 9-inch (33 x 23 cm) baking dish with enough freezer wrap to generously cover bottom, sides, and overlap the top. Spray with cooking spray. Spread grits in dish. Top with onion and mushroom mixture. Seal freezer wrap. Freeze until solid and then remove baking dish.

## TO REHEAT

Let individual servings thaw in refrigerator overnight. For large portion, remove freezer wrap and place in 13 x 9-inch (33 x 23 cm) baking dish before thawing in refrigerator.

MICROWAVE METHOD: Reheat individual servings in the microwave on high for 2 minutes or until heated through.

OVEN METHOD: Preheat oven to 350°F (180°C, or gas mark 4). Cover baking dish with foil and bake for 20 minutes. Uncover and bake 10 more minutes.

AMOUNT PER SERVING: Calories 592.79; Total Fat 19.99 g; Cholesterol 39.53 mg; Sodium 325.47 mg; Potassium 1696.79 mg; Total Carbohydrates 97.4 g; Fiber 13.73 g; Sugar 3.72 g; Protein 19.46 g

# FABULOUSLY LOW-FAT BAKED FALAFELS

Traditionally a high-fat fried food, falafels can be made with scrumptiously flavorful ingredients and baked for a filling, yet low-fat, vegetarian meal. Tuck falafels into pitas drizzled with a tzatziki sauce or let the kids dip their falafels in a tahini sauce or low-fat ranch.

..............................................................................................................................................

**1 cup (120 g) cracked wheat or (100 g) bulgur**

**2 cups (475 ml) boiling water**

**2 cans (15 ounces, or 425 g, each) garbanzo beans, rinsed, drained**

**1 small red onion, finely chopped**

**½ cup (8 g) finely chopped fresh cilantro**

**3 cloves garlic, crushed**

**1 tablespoon (15 ml) olive oil**

**3 eggs, lightly beaten**

**1½ tablespoons (9 g) cumin seed, toasted and ground**

**1½ tablespoons (8 g) coriander seed, toasted and ground**

**1 teaspoon salt**

**Freshly ground black pepper to taste**

**Pinch of cayenne pepper**

**Juice and grated zest of 1 small lemon**

① In a medium bowl, combine bulgur and water. Seal and set aside until water is absorbed or grains are tender.

② In a food processor, combine beans, onion, cilantro, garlic, oil, eggs, cumin, coriander, salt, black pepper, cayenne, and lemon juice and zest. Pulse to combine. Drain excess water from bulgur, squeezing if necessary. Add to garbanzo mixture and pulse until well-combined.

③ Preheat oven to 400°F (200°C, or gas mark 6). Shape garbanzo mixture into 12 patties. Spray both sides generously with olive oil or cooking spray. Place on a baking sheet and bake for 8 minutes. Flip and spray with oil again. Bake for 8 minutes or until heated through. Let cool completely.

YIELD: 12 FALAFELS, OR 12 SERVINGS

## NUTRITION SPOTLIGHT: GARBANZO BEANS

Low in fat, high in fiber, and ultra-nutritious, canned garbanzo beans (chickpeas) are a kitchen must-have. Here are some of my favorite ways to use them:

- Puréed with olive oil, garlic, and fresh herbs for hummus.
- Puréed and used as the base of a soup or use as part of the fat in baked goods.
- Tossed into salads, soups, stews, and chili.
- Tossed with kidney beans, green beans, sliced red onions, and vinaigrette.

 TO FREEZE

INDIVIDUAL SERVINGS: Wrap each falafel in freezer wrap and place in a large freezer bag.

FOR A CROWD: Set falafels on a baking sheet and freeze until solid. Transfer to a large freezer bag or freezer-safe container.

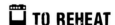 TO REHEAT

Let falafels thaw in the refrigerator for a few hours.

MICROWAVE METHOD: Falafels won't be crispy if microwaved, but they will be just as flavorful. Reheat individual falafels on high for 1 to 2 minutes or until heated through.

OVEN METHOD: Preheat oven to 375°F (190°C, or gas mark 5). Place falafels on a baking sheet and bake for 10 minutes. Heat broiler and broil falafels 2 minutes on each side or until lightly crisped.

AMOUNT PER SERVING: Calories 172.87; Total Fat 3.69 g; Cholesterol 52.88 mg; Sodium 428 mg; Potassium 232.53 mg; Total Carbohydrates 29.36 g; Fiber 6.35 g; Sugar 0.3 g; Protein 7.27 g

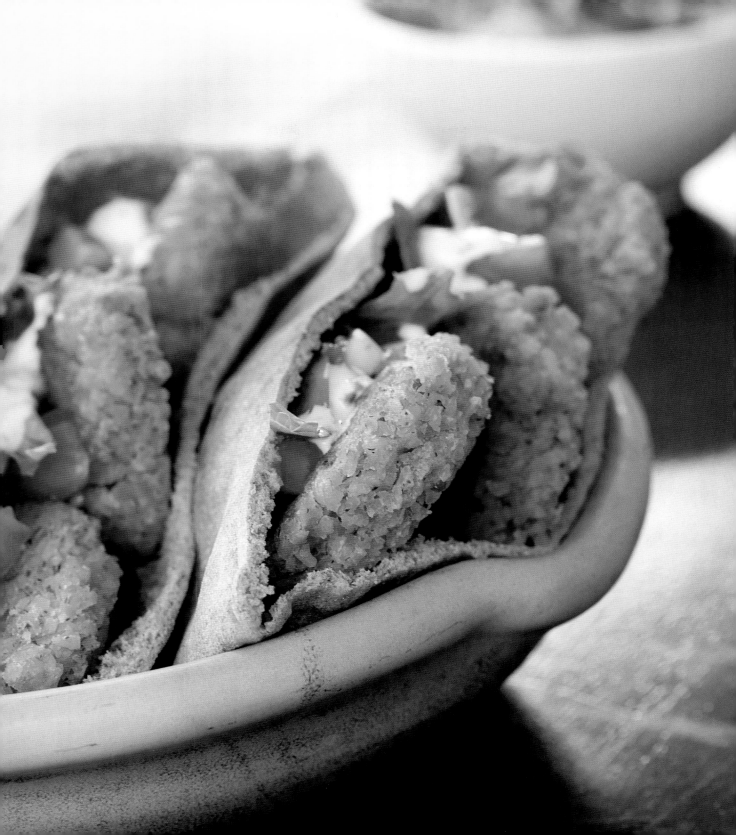

# VEGETARIAN TERIYAKI STIR-FRY

A medley of crisp, tender vegetables in a flavorful Asian sauce, this dish is loaded with vitamins, minerals, antioxidants, and other health-promoting phytonutrients. For a meat-eating change, add shrimp, strips of lean beef or pork, or skinless chicken breast or thighs.

.....................................................................................................................

1 cup (235 ml) tamari

¾ cup (255 g) honey

1 cup (235 ml) mirin

½ cup (120 ml) orange juice

3 tablespoons (18 g) minced fresh ginger

2 cloves garlic, minced

1 tablespoon (8 g) All-Purpose Asian Spice Blend (page 174) (optional)

2 tablespoons (28 ml) canola oil

2 cups (244 g) thinly sliced carrots

1 onion, halved, thinly sliced

2 cups (142 g) broccoli florets, sliced

2 cups (200 g) cauliflower florets, sliced

1 large red bell pepper, seeded, sliced

1 pound (455 g) sliced mushrooms

1 can (11 ounces, 310 g) mandarin oranges, drained

1 cup (110 g) sliced almonds, toasted

6 to 8 cups (684 g to 912 g) steamed brown rice or cooked soba noodles cooked just to al dente

① In a medium saucepan over medium heat, combine tamari, honey, mirin, orange juice, ginger, garlic, and Asian Spice Blend. Cook, stirring, until mixture comes to a boil. Remove from heat and set aside.

② Heat oil in a large wok over medium-high heat. Add carrots, onion, broccoli, and cauliflower and stir-fry until vegetables are just starting to get tender. Add bell pepper and mushrooms and stir-fry until peppers are tender and mushrooms have released their liquid.

③ Add 1 cup (235 ml) of teriyaki sauce to wok and toss to coat vegetables. Add more sauce, if desired. Remove from heat and let vegetables and sauce cool completely. Stir in mandarin oranges and almonds.

YIELD: 8 SERVINGS

 ## TO FREEZE

INDIVIDUAL SERVINGS: Divide rice or noodles among 8 freezer- and microwave-safe containers. Toss stir-fry to distribute sauce and add to containers. Freeze leftover sauce in an ice cube tray.

FOR A CROWD: Transfer rice or noodles to a large freezer bag. Toss stir-fry to distribute sauce and transfer to a large freezer bag, removing as much air as possible before sealing. Transfer leftover sauce to a 1-quart (950 ml) freezer bag.

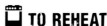 ## TO REHEAT

Let rice, stir-fry, and sauce thaw overnight in the refrigerator.

MICROWAVE METHOD: Reheat individual servings of stir-fry in the microwave on high for 2 to 3 minutes or until heated through, stirring every minute. Add thawed sauce before or after reheating.

STOVETOP METHOD: Reheat stir-fry in a wok over medium-high heat, stirring often, adding oil or water for moisture, if needed. Reheat rice or noodles in a saucepan over medium heat. Sprinkle with a little water and toss until heated through.

AMOUNT PER SERVING: Calories 312.01; Total Fat 11.74 g; Cholesterol 0 mg; Sodium 171.09 mg; Potassium 629.01 mg; Total Carbohydrates 45.5 g; Fiber 7.17 g; Sugar 9.11 g; Protein 10.04 g

# RED LENTIL AND COUSCOUS VEGGIE BURGERS  *Try*

What kid doesn't love a burger? Introducing veggie burgers into your children's diet now will expand their burger loving from meat-only to other meatless—and tasty—alternatives. Your kids can even help mix and shape these lentil burgers and choose their own toppings for dinner.

6 ounces (170 g) dried red lentils

2 tablespoons (28 ml) olive oil

1 onion, minced

1 red bell pepper, seeded, minced

1 clove garlic, minced

½ cup (75 g) dried currants, rehydrated in orange juice

1 cup (175 g) whole-wheat couscous, cooked

¼ cup (36 g) sunflower seeds

Salt and freshly ground black pepper

2 eggs, beaten

8 whole-grain hamburger buns

① Cook lentils according to package directions, drain, and set aside to cool. While lentils are cooling, heat oil in a skillet and cook onion and bell pepper, stirring often, until very tender. Add garlic and cook, stirring, for 1 minute. Remove from heat.

② Drain currants and stir them into the onion mixture. Transfer mixture to a large bowl to cool. Add lentils, couscous, and sunflower seeds, using your hands to combine. Taste and season with salt and pepper.

③ Mix egg into the lentil mixture, cover bowl, and refrigerate for 30 minutes. Turn on oven broiler. Divide lentil mixture into 8 patties.

④ Spray patties with cooking spray on both sides or brush both sides with olive oil. Broil for 3 to 4 minutes, flip, and broil second side for 3 to 4 minutes or until lightly browned. Let cool completely.

YIELD: 8 BURGERS, OR 8 SERVINGS

##  TO FREEZE

INDIVIDUAL SERVINGS: Wrap each patty in freezer wrap and place in a large freezer bag. Wrap each bun in freezer wrap and place in a second large freezer bag.

FOR A CROWD: Place patties on a baking sheet and freeze until solid. Place patties in a large freezer bag, removing as much air as possible before sealing. Place buns on a baking sheet and freeze until solid and then freeze in a large freezer bag, removing as much air as possible before sealing.

##  TO REHEAT

Let burgers thaw in the refrigerator overnight. Let buns thaw at room temperature for a couple of hours; toast buns if desired.

MICROWAVE METHOD: Individual patties can be reheated in the microwave on high for 1 to 2 minutes or until heated through. Serve on whole-grain buns and with your choice of toppings.

OVEN METHOD: Preheat oven to 375°F (190°C, or gas mark 5). Place patties on a greased baking sheet and bake for 12 minutes or until heated through. Serve on whole-grain buns and with your choice of toppings.

AMOUNT PER SERVING: Calories 220; Total Fat 0 g; Cholesterol 0 mg; Sodium 5 mg; Total Carbohydrates 44 g; Fiber 7 g; Sugar 4 g; Protein 8 g

# CHAPTER 7

# BREADS, ROLLS, PIZZAS, AND MORE

## WHOLE GRAINS NEVER TASTED SO GOOD

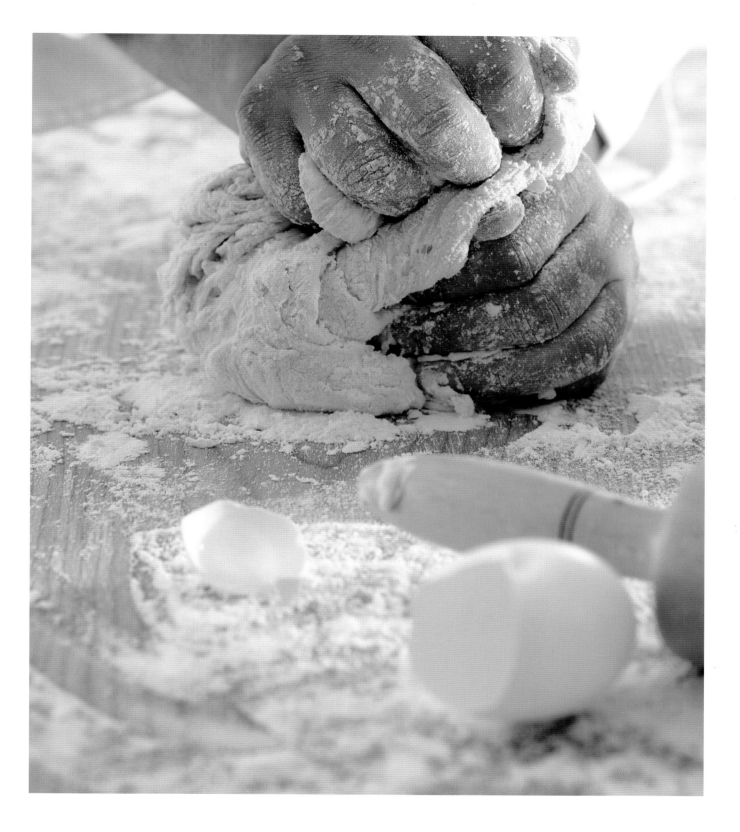

# ZESTY GARLIC-ROSEMARY BREAD

There's more to bread than buying a bagged loaf in the supermarket bread aisle. Though convenient, many mass-produced breads are laden with additives, preservatives, unhealthy fats, and sugar. Baking bread at home is not only cost-effective, but you can also feel good about feeding your family a wholesome loaf. Are you intimidated by yeast-risen breads? This recipe is as easy as they come. The result is a fragrant, hearty bread perfect for sandwiches, dipping in olive oil, croutons, and even Whole-Grain Bread Crumbs (page 175).

½ cup (120 ml) warm water

2 teaspoons granulated sugar

1 tablespoon (12 g) dry active yeast

1 can (12 ounces, or 355 ml) evaporated milk

2 tablespoons (28 ml) extra-virgin olive oil

1½ teaspoons salt

2½ cups (300 g) whole-wheat flour

2½ to 3 cups (313 to 375 g) all-purpose flour

2 tablespoons (4 g) coarsely chopped fresh rosemary

4 cloves garlic, minced

Grated zest of 1 large lemon

① Place water in the bowl of a standup mixer fitted with the dough hook attachment. Sprinkle sugar and yeast over water and set aside for 10 minutes or until mixture becomes frothy.

② Add milk, olive oil, salt, and whole-wheat flour. Turn mixer on medium and mix until combined. Add 2½ cups (313 g) all-purpose flour, rosemary, garlic, and lemon zest. Mix on medium-low until flour is incorporated and then turn speed up to medium-high. Knead with dough hook for 8 minutes or until a soft dough forms and pulls away from the bowl. Add a bit more flour if mixture is still sticky.

③ Dump dough onto a lightly floured surface and knead into a ball. Rub a large bowl with olive oil. Place dough in bowl, turning over to coat with olive oil. Cover with a damp towel. Set in a warm, draft-free area and let rise for 1 hour or until doubled in size.

④ Rub two 8 x 4-inch (20 x 10 cm) loaf pans with olive oil and set aside. Punch dough down and dump onto a lightly floured surface. Divide in half and shape each into a loaf. Place each in a loaf pan and set in a warm, draft-free area. Cover with a damp towel and let rise for 45 minutes or until doubled in size.

⑤ Meanwhile, preheat oven to 425°F (220°C, or gas mark 7). Use a sharp knife to slash the tops of the loaves. Bake for 10 minutes. Reduce oven heat to 325°F (170°C, or gas mark 3) and continue baking for 15 minutes or until bread is lightly browned and sounds hollow when tapped. Remove from pans and cool completely on a wire rack.

YIELD: 2 LOAVES, OR 32 SERVINGS

Amount Per Serving:Calories 102.28; Total Fat 2.03 g; Cholesterol 3.43 mg; Sodium 122.65 mg; Potassium 102.6 mg; Total Carbohydrates 18.16 g; Fiber 1.77 g; Sugar 1.54 g; Protein 3.57 g

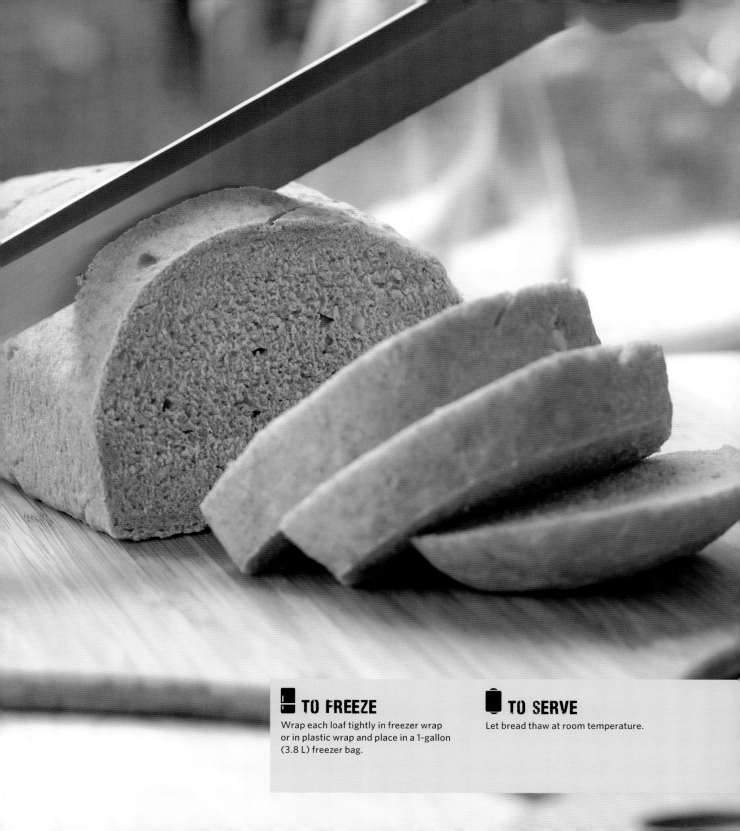

## TO FREEZE
Wrap each loaf tightly in freezer wrap or in plastic wrap and place in a 1-gallon (3.8 L) freezer bag.

## TO SERVE
Let bread thaw at room temperature.

# WHOLE-GRAIN SEEDED BREAD

Studded with a medley of crunchy seeds, this hearty bread is healthy goodness with every bite. In addition to the good-for-you whole grains, the seeds are loaded with heart-healthy unsaturated fats.

......................................................................................................................................................

**1½ cups (150 g) whole-wheat flour**

**1 cup (125 g) all-purpose flour**

**¾ cup (60 g) rolled oats**

**2 tablespoons (14 g) ground flaxseed**

**⅓ cup (48 g) sunflower seeds**

**⅓ cup (76 g) pumpkin seeds**

**2 tablespoons (16 g) sesame seeds**

**2 tablespoons (18 g) poppy seeds**

**1 tablespoon (12 g) dry active yeast**

**1½ teaspoons salt**

**2 tablespoons (16 g) vital wheat gluten**

**1½ cups (355 ml) warm water**

**¼ cup (85 g) brown rice syrup**

**¼ cup (60 ml) olive oil**

**Cornmeal for sprinkling**

**Seeds for sprinkling**

① In the bowl of a standup mixer fitted with the paddle attachment, combine flours, oats, flax, seeds, yeast, salt, and vital wheat gluten.

② In a small bowl, whisk together water, brown rice syrup, and oil. Add to flour mixture and blend on low until well-combined, scraping down the sides of the bowl occasionally. Increase speed to medium and knead for 7 to 8 minutes. Dump onto a lightly floured surface and shape into a ball.

③ Rub a large bowl with olive oil. Place dough in bowl, turning it over to coat with oil. Cover with a damp towel and set in a warm, draft-free area. Allow to rise for 1½ hours or until doubled in size. Punch dough down and dump it onto a lightly floured surface.

④ Divide dough in half and shape each half into a ball. Set on a pizza peel sprinkled with cornmeal. Cover with plastic wrap and allow to rise for 45 minutes.

⑤ Meanwhile, place a pizza stone on the middle rack in the oven and preheat to 400°F (200°C, or gas mark 6). Place a large baking pan on the bottom rack and fill with 1 to 2 cups (235 to 475 ml) of hot water. Brush bread with water, slash the top with a sharp knife, and sprinkle with seeds. Slide bread onto pizza stone.

⑥ Bake for 40 minutes or until bread sounds hollow when tapped. Remove from oven and set on a wire rack to cool completely.

YIELD: 2 LOAVES, OR 32 SERVINGS

## COOKING TIP: TEST YOUR YEAST

If you use expired or old yeast, your baked goods are going to literally and figuratively fall flat. To test active dry yeast, sprinkle a scant 1 teaspoon over a ½ cup (120 ml) of warm water and 1 teaspoon sugar. Active yeast will expand and become bubbly or foamy in a few minutes. If your yeast barely forms a foam or does nothing at all, it's dead and needs to be discarded.

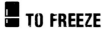 **TO FREEZE**

Wrap each loaf tightly in freezer wrap or in plastic wrap and place in a 1-gallon (3.8 L) freezer bag.

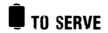 **TO SERVE**

Let bread thaw at room temperature.

AMOUNT PER SERVING: Calories 101.1; Total Fat 4.34 g; Cholesterol 0 mg; Sodium 24.56 mg; Potassium 87.67 mg; Total Carbohydrates 22.53 g; Fiber 1.53 g; Sugar 0.22 g; Protein 3.08 g

# HONEY WHOLE-WHEAT FREEZER ROLLS

Warm, fresh-from-the-oven rolls are the perfect accompaniment for salads, soups, and juicy meat and poultry dishes as well as a tasty choice for sliders or mini sandwiches. In addition to tasting bakery-fresh, the hint of honey and the whole-wheat flour give these rolls a healthy edge compared to the packaged freezer rolls from the supermarket. You won't find any artificial flavorings or additives in this recipe.

**¾ cup (175 ml) warm water, divided**

**1 packet (2¼ teaspoons, or 9 g) active dry yeast**

**¼ cup (60 ml) warm milk**

**3 tablespoons (42 g) unsalted butter, softened at room temperature**

**3 tablespoons (60 g) honey**

**1 teaspoon salt**

**2½ to 3 cups (300 to 375 g) whole-wheat flour, divided**

**1 egg**

①  Place ¼ cup (60 ml) warm water in the bowl of a standup mixer fitted with the paddle attachment. Sprinkle in yeast; stir until dissolved.

②  Add remaining water, warm milk, butter, honey, salt, and 1 cup (120 g) flour. Beat on medium speed until well-combined.

③  Add egg and ½ cup (60 g) flour, mixing until well-combined. Switch to the dough hook and add remaining flour. Knead dough on medium-high speed for 7 to 8 minutes or until dough is smooth and elastic. Dump onto a lightly floured surface and form into a ball.

④  Grease a large bowl and place dough in bowl, turning to coat with oil. Cover with a damp towel and set in a warm, draft-free place. Let dough rise for about 30 minutes.

⑤  Punch dough down and dump onto a lightly floured surface. Divide dough into 12 equal pieces and roll into balls.

YIELD: 12 ROLLS, OR 12 SERVINGS

 **TO FREEZE**

Place rolls on a greased baking sheet and place in freezer until solid. Transfer rolls to a freezer bag, removing as much air as possible before sealing.

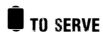 **TO SERVE**

Remove desired amount of rolls from freezer and place them on a greased baking sheet. Cover with plastic and set in a warm, draft-free place. Let rise until doubled in size, about 1¼ hours.

OVEN METHOD: Bake at 350°F (180°C or gas mark 4) for 15 minutes or until lightly browned and baked through.

AMOUNT PER SERVING:  Calories 156.98; Total Fat 3.97 g; Cholesterol 25.56 mg; Sodium 204.7 mg; Potassium 158.51 mg; Total Carbohydrates 27.36 g; Fiber 3.98 g; Sugar 4.53 g; Protein 5.31 g

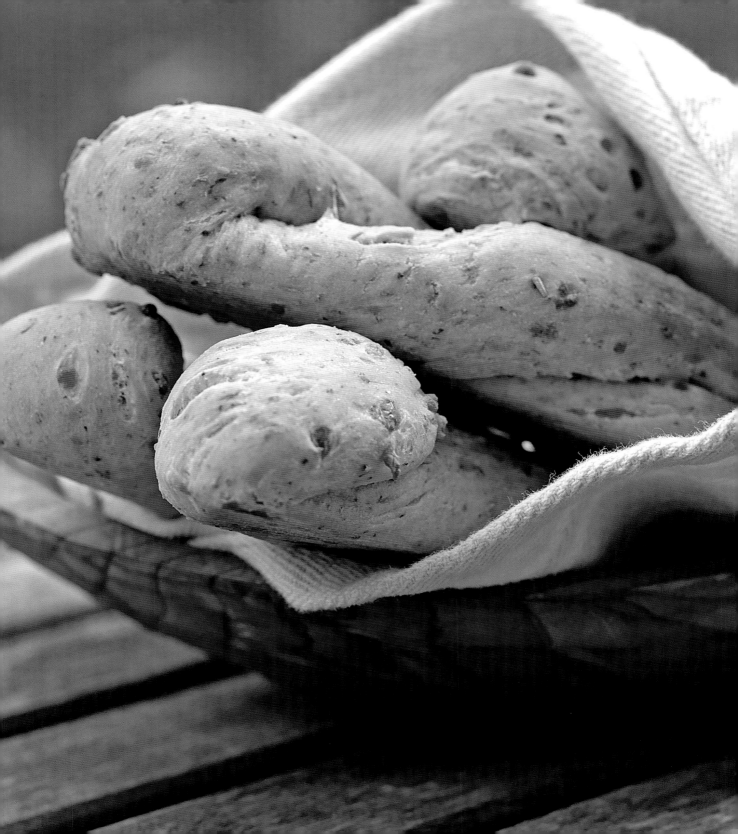

# WHOLE-GRAIN PARMESAN HERB TWISTS

Homemade bread twists are not only impressive to serve to dinner guests, but they are a fun kid-friendly accompaniment to dinner, particularly Three-Bean Italian Minestrone Soup (page 95). Their flavorful whole-grain goodness also partners well with green salads tossed in a tangy balsamic vinaigrette.

¾ cup (175 ml) warm water

1 packet (2¼ teaspoons, or 9 g) active dry yeast

¼ cup (60 ml) warm milk

3 tablespoons (42 g) unsalted butter, softened at room temperature

2 tablespoons (40 g) honey

1 teaspoon salt

2 cups (240 g) whole-wheat flour, divided

1 egg

1 cup (125 g) all-purpose flour

½ cup (40 g) shredded Parmesan cheese

1 tablespoon (6 g) Italian seasoning

① Place ¼ cup (60 ml) warm water in the bowl of a standup mixer fitted with the paddle attachment. Sprinkle in yeast; stir until dissolved.

② Add remaining water, warm milk, butter, honey, salt, and 1 cup (120 g) whole-wheat flour. Beat on medium speed until well-combined.

③ Add egg and ½ cup (60 g) whole-wheat flour, mixing until well-combined. Switch to the dough hook and add remaining whole-wheat flour, all-purpose flour, cheese, and seasoning. Knead dough on medium-high speed for 7 to 8 minutes or until dough is smooth and elastic. Dump onto a lightly floured surface and form into a ball.

④ Grease a large bowl and place dough in bowl, turning to coat with oil. Cover with a damp towel and set in a warm, draft-free place. Let dough rise for about 30 minutes.

⑤ Punch dough down and dump onto a lightly floured surface. Divide dough into 12 equal pieces and roll each into a 10-inch (25 cm) rope. Fold each rope in half and pinch the ends together. Twist each rope three times.

YIELD: 12 TWISTS, OR 12 SERVINGS

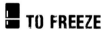 **TO FREEZE**

Place twists on a greased baking sheet and place in freezer just until solid. Transfer to a freezer bag, removing as much air as possible before sealing.

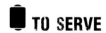 **TO SERVE**

Remove desired number of twists from freezer and place them on a greased baking sheet. Cover with plastic and set in a warm, draft-free place. Let rise until doubled in size, about 1¼ hours.

OVEN METHOD: Bake at 350°F (180°C, or gas mark 4) for 15 minutes or until lightly browned and baked through.

AMOUNT PER SERVING: Calories 169.28; Total Fat 4.85 g; Cholesterol 28.5 mg; Sodium 255.35 mg; Potassium 130.77 mg; Total Carbohydrates 26.6 g; Fiber 3.01 g; Sugar 3.18 g; Protein 6.25 g

# BUTTERMILK CORN BREAD

Better than a box mix, this moist, mouthwatering corn bread features the zing of jalapeño and the sweet hint of honey. Keeping a double or triple batch in the freezer gives you a convenient accompaniment for salads, soups, and stews, as well as a whole-grain base for holiday stuffing.

6 tablespoons (90 ml) canola oil

2 cups (320 g) finely chopped onion

2 jalapeños, halved, seeded, minced

¼ cup (4 g) minced fresh cilantro

2½ cups (345 g) yellow cornmeal

2 cups (240 g) whole-wheat pastry flour

4 teaspoons (18.4 g) baking powder

1 teaspoon (4.6 g) baking soda

1 teaspoon salt

2 eggs

2½ cups (570 ml) buttermilk

¼ cup (85 g) honey

1. Preheat oven to 400°F (200°C, or gas mark 6). Grease two 8-inch (20 cm) baking dishes.

2. Heat oil in a small skillet over medium-high heat. Cook onion and jalapeños, stirring often, for 5 minutes. Stir in cilantro and remove from heat.

3. In a large bowl, whisk together cornmeal, flour, baking powder, baking soda, and salt. In a small bowl, whisk together eggs, buttermilk, and honey. Stir onion mixture into buttermilk mixture. Add buttermilk mixture to flour mixture, stirring until just combined.

4. Pour batter into prepared pans and bake for 20 minutes or until a cake tester inserted in the center comes out clean. Cool in pan for 10 minutes. Invert onto a wire rack and cool completely.

YIELD: TWO 8-INCH (20 CM) BREADS, OR 12 SERVINGS

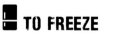 TO FREEZE

Wrap each tightly in freezer wrap.

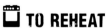 TO REHEAT

Let thaw at room temperature.

OVEN METHOD: Preheat oven to 350°F (180°C, or gas mark 4). Place corn bread in a baking dish and bake for 10 minutes or until warmed.

AMOUNT PER SERVING: Calories 305.56; Total Fat 9.8 g; Cholesterol 37.22 mg; Sodium 849.44 mg; Potassium 333.46 mg; Total Carbohydrates 49.3 g; Fiber 5.61 g; Sugar 10.04 g; Protein 8.36 g

# SECRETLY WHOLESOME SOFT PRETZELS

Chewy, soft whole-grain pretzels dipped in mustard or a low-fat creamy dressing are a tasty, healthy, after-school treat for hungry kids.

1½ cups (355 ml) warm water

1 tablespoon (20 g) honey

2 teaspoons (8 g) active dry yeast

1 teaspoon salt

2 cups (240 g) whole-wheat flour, divided

2 cups (250 g) all-purpose flour

Coarse-grain kosher salt

①  In the bowl of a standup mixer fitted with the paddle attachment, stir together water, honey, and yeast on low speed for 30 seconds. Set aside for 5 to 6 minutes or until bubbly. Stir in salt and 1 cup (120 g) whole-wheat flour on low speed until combined.

②  Add remaining whole-wheat flour and all-purpose flour 1 cup (125 g) at a time and blend on low until just combined. Switch to dough hook and knead on medium-high speed for 7 to 8 minutes or until dough is smooth and elastic.

③  Grease a large bowl. Dump dough onto a lightly floured surface and knead into a ball. Place in bowl, turning to coat with oil. Cover with a damp towel and set in a warm, draft-free place. Let rise for 1 hour.

④  Punch dough down and transfer to a lightly floured surface. Divide into 16 pieces and roll each piece into thick ropes. Shape ropes into pretzels. Place on a greased baking sheet and cover with plastic. Let rise for 30 minutes.

⑤  Preheat oven to 425°F (220°C, or gas mark 7). Bring a large pot of water to a boil. Boil pretzels for 3 to 4 minutes, turning once. Transfer to a wire rack to drain. Arrange pretzels on a baking sheet, sprinkle with kosher salt, and bake for 15 minutes or until just turning golden. Transfer to wire racks to cool completely.

YIELD: 16 PRETZELS, OR 16 SERVINGS

*Recipe continued on next page*

AMOUNT PER SERVING:  Calories 115.12; Total Fat 0.47 g; Cholesterol 0 mg; Sodium 147.4 mg; Potassium 90.9 mg; Total Carbohydrates 24.48 g; Fiber 2.44 g; Sugar 1.13 g; Protein 3.95 g

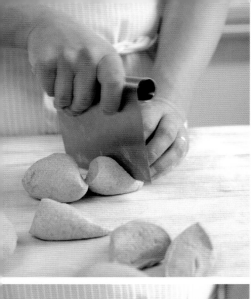
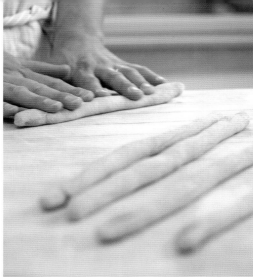
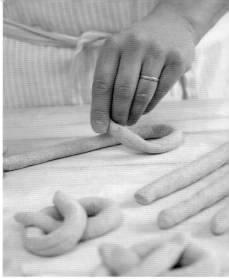
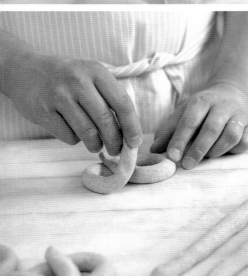
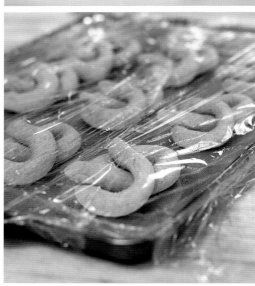
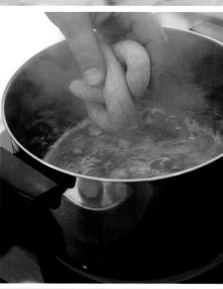
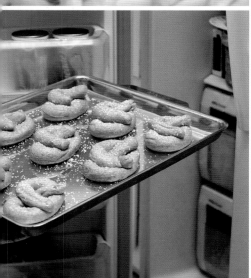

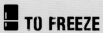

## ▣ TO FREEZE

Place baking sheet in freezer until pretzels are solid. Transfer to a large freezer bag or container.

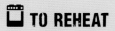

## ▣ TO REHEAT

MICROWAVE METHOD: Place frozen pretzel in microwave on 60% power for 2 to 3 minutes or until soft and warm.

OVEN METHOD: Preheat oven to 400°F (200°C, or gas mark 6). Bake pretzels for 5 to 6 minutes or until soft and warm.

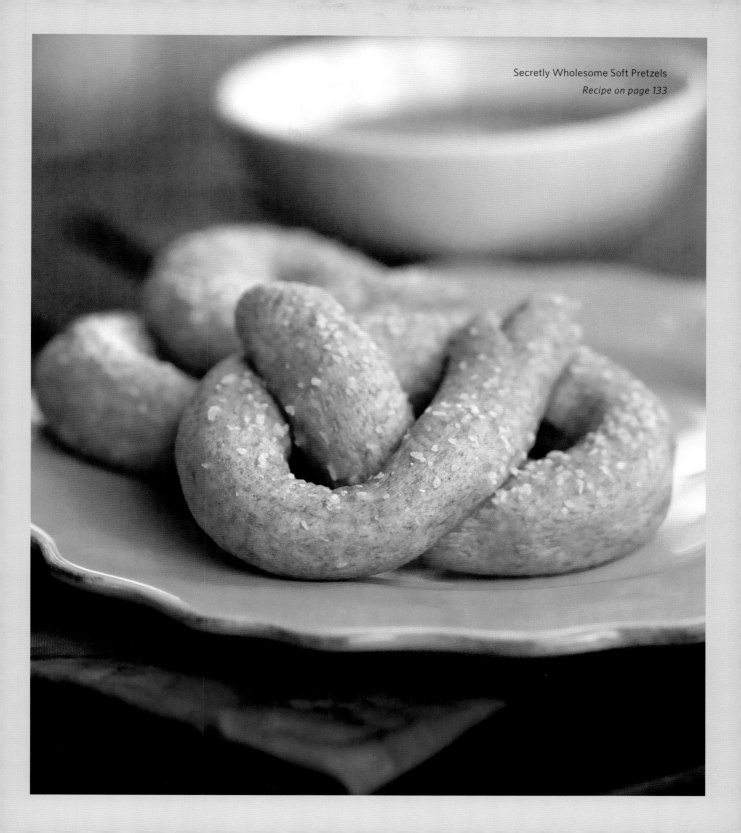
Secretly Wholesome Soft Pretzels
*Recipe on page 133*

# QUICK KALAMATA OLIVE AND ROSEMARY SCONES

A scrumptious change from bread, rice, or pasta, savory scones are a welcome accompaniment for braised beef, Zesty Marinated Lamb Chops (page 55), roasted chicken, and steamy stews or Three-Bean Italian Minestrone Soup (page 95). Deliciously studded with kalamata olives, fresh rosemary, and feta cheese, these Mediterranean-inspired scones are also an irresistible snack.

1 cup (125 g) all-purpose flour

¾ cup (90 g) whole-wheat pastry flour

2½ teaspoons (11.5 g) baking powder

Pinch of salt

A few grinds of black pepper

½ cup (112 g) unsalted butter, chilled, cut into small pieces

½ cup (75 g) crumbled feta cheese

½ cup (85 g) pitted kalamata olives, chopped

1 clove garlic, minced

2 teaspoons minced fresh rosemary

½ cup (115 g) plain Greek yogurt

4 tablespoons (60 ml) milk, divided

① Preheat oven to 400°F (200°C, or gas mark 6). In a large bowl, whisk together flours, baking powder, salt, and pepper.

② Add butter to flour mixture and use your fingers or a pastry cutter to blend butter into flour mixture to form a coarse meal. Stir in cheese, olives, garlic, and rosemary.

③ In a small bowl, whisk together yogurt and 2 tablespoons (28 ml) milk. Add to flour mixture and stir until dough comes together. Dump dough onto a lightly floured surface. Gently knead a few times and form a flat disk. Cut into 8 wedges.

④ Place wedges on a baking sheet and brush lightly with remaining milk. Bake for 25 minutes or until just golden. Transfer to a wire rack to cool completely.

YIELD: 8 SCONES, OR 8 SERVINGS

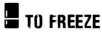 **TO FREEZE**

Place scones on a baking sheet and freeze until solid. Tightly wrap individual scones in freezer wrap or place multiple scones in 1-gallon (3.8 L) freezer bags.

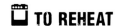 **TO REHEAT**

Let scones come to room temperature.

OVEN METHOD: Preheat oven to 350°F (180°C, or gas mark 4). Place scones on a baking sheet and warm in oven for 5 to 8 minutes or until heated through.

AMOUNT PER SERVING: Calories 253.1; Total Fat 15.76 g; Cholesterol 39.93 mg; Sodium 408.45 mg; Potassium 122.95 mg; Total Carbohydrates 23.24 g; Fiber 1.92 g; Sugar 1.89 g; Protein 5.73 g

# FAST AND EASY FRESH HERB FOCACCIA

Whole-wheat focaccia can be served as a hearty accompaniment for salads and soups or for sandwiches.

........................................................................................................................

**2½ teaspoons (10 g) active dry yeast**

**1 cup (235 ml) warm water, divided**

**1 tablespoon (20 g) honey**

**2 tablespoons (28 ml) extra-virgin olive oil plus more for brushing**

**1 cup (125 g) all-purpose flour plus more for kneading**

**1 teaspoon salt**

**1 cup (120 g) whole-wheat flour**

**2 teaspoons finely chopped fresh rosemary**

**1 tablespoon (4 g) minced fresh parsley**

**1 tablespoon (2 g) fresh thyme leaves**

**2 tablespoons (2 g) finely chopped fresh chives**

**Coarse salt**

① In the bowl of a standup mixer fitted with the dough hook, stir together yeast, ¼ cup (60 ml) water, and honey. Let stand for 10 minutes or until yeast has bloomed and is frothy.

② Add remaining water, olive oil, all-purpose flour, and salt, mixing until smooth. Add whole-wheat flour, rosemary, parsley, thyme, and chives. With mixer on low, mix until dough comes together.

③ Increase mixer speed to medium-high and knead for about 8 minutes or until dough is smooth and elastic. Dump dough onto a lightly floured surface and knead into a ball.

④ Wipe a large bowl with olive oil and place dough in bowl, turning to coat. Cover with a damp towel and place bowl in a warm, draft-free place. Let rise for 1½ hours or until doubled in size. Punch dough down and dump it onto a lightly floured surface. Divide dough in two.

⑤ Lightly oil two 8-inch (20 cm) baking pans. Stretch each portion of dough to fit in the pans with an even thickness. If dough is difficult to work with, cover it with a slightly damp towel and let it sit for 10 minutes.

⑥ Cover pans with kitchen towels and set in a warm place for 45 minutes or until doubled in size. Preheat oven to 475°F (240°C, or gas mark 9). Use your fingers to indent the dough in several places. Cover pans with towels and let rise for another 15 minutes.

⑦ Bake for 15 to 18 minutes or until focaccia is baked through and golden. Brush the tops with olive oil and sprinkle with coarse salt. Remove from pans and let cool completely on wire racks.

YIELD: TWO 8-INCH (20 CM) FOCACCIA, OR 12 SERVINGS

## SERVING SUGGESTIONS

Here are five must-try focaccia sandwich combinations:

- Roasted peppers, spinach leaves, red onions, provolone, and a light mayo or aioli with a pinch of cayenne
- Light mayo, thin slices of roast beef and Havarti, and Best-by-the-Batch Caramelized Onions (page 104)
- Toasted Almond and Basil Pesto (page 169), roasted turkey, sun-dried tomatoes, and feta crumbles
- Prosciutto, Roma tomatoes, fresh mozzarella, basil leaves, olive oil, and balsamic vinegar
- Turkey, shaved Parmesan, cranberry sauce, and radicchio

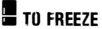 **TO FREEZE**

INDIVIDUAL SERVINGS: Cut each focaccia into 6 pieces and wrap with freezer wrap.

FOR A CROWD: Wrap each focaccia in freezer wrap.

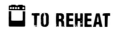 **TO REHEAT**

Let focaccia thaw at room temperature for a few hours.

MICROWAVE METHOD: Reheat individual servings on high for 20 to 30 seconds.

OVEN METHOD: Preheat oven to 350°F (180°C, or gas mark 4). Place whole focaccia in original baking pans and bake for 10 to 15 minutes or until heated through.

AMOUNT PER SERVING: Calories 100.46; Total Fat 2.49 g; Cholesterol 0 mg; Sodium 195.97 mg; Potassium 75.87 mg; Total Carbohydrates 17.38 g; Fiber 1.84 g; Sugar 1.45 g; Protein 2.86 g

# WHOLE-GRAIN PIZZA DOUGH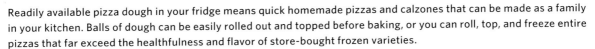

Readily available pizza dough in your fridge means quick homemade pizzas and calzones that can be made as a family in your kitchen. Balls of dough can be easily rolled out and topped before baking, or you can roll, top, and freeze entire pizzas that far exceed the healthfulness and flavor of store-bought frozen varieties.

3 tablespoons (36 g) yeast

3 cups (700 ml) warm water

2 tablespoons (26 g) granulated sugar

4 cups (480 g) whole-wheat flour

4 cups (500 g) all-purpose flour

3 teaspoons (18 g) salt

1½ tablespoons (5 g) dried oregano

¼ cup (60 ml) extra-virgin olive oil

① In a large bowl, combine yeast, water, and sugar. Let sit for 10 minutes to bloom yeast.

② Add flours, salt, oregano, and olive oil. Stir until ingredients come together. Dump onto a lightly floured surface and knead for about 10 minutes or until dough becomes elastic, adding more flour a bit at a time if dough is too sticky.

③ Place dough in a well-oiled very large bowl, turning dough to coat with oil. Cover with a damp kitchen towel and place bowl in a warm, draft-free place. Let rise for 1 hour or until doubled in size.

④ Punch dough down and dump onto a lightly floured surface. Divide into 4 portions and roll out each portion into a 10-inch (25 cm) round.

YIELD: 4 PIZZAS, OR 32 SERVINGS

## SERVING SUGGESTIONS

Here are just a few of the tasty ways you can put pizza dough to work:

- Family-size pizzas to feed a hungry crowd (each portion of dough will serve 8)
- Individual-size pizzas perfect for pleasing picky eaters (each portion will make 6 to 8 small pizzas)
- Mini pizzas to serve as awesome appetizers (each portion will make 16 to 20 mini pizzas)
- Calzones (each portion will make 3 or 4 calzones)

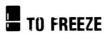 TO FREEZE

Tightly wrap crusts with plastic wrap and then heavy-duty foil.

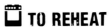 TO REHEAT

Let dough thaw overnight in the refrigerator.

OVEN METHOD: Place a pizza stone in the oven and preheat oven to 425°F (220°C, or gas mark 7). Top crust with your favorite toppings. Place pizza on a pizza stone. Bake for 10 to 12 minutes or until crust is golden and cheese is melted.

AMOUNT PER SERVING: Calories 131.87; Total Fat 2.22 g; Cholesterol 0 mg; Sodium 220.39 mg; Potassium 105.15 mg; Total Carbohydrates 24.6 g; Fiber 2.62 g; Sugar 0.92 g; Protein 4.2 g

# MEDITERRANEAN VEGGIE LOVER'S PIZZA

Veggies and feta piled on a whole-grain crust make one tasty meat-free meal. This is a simple pizza recipe that has many variations, depending on the vegetables in season and the types of cheese you have on hand. Make a variety of veggie pizzas to keep in your freezer, and you'll always have a meatless alternative to serve to your family or for vegetarian guests.

**2 portions fresh Whole-Grain Pizza Dough (page 138)**

**Vegetable shortening**

**2 tablespoons (28 ml) olive oil**

**1½ cups (240 g) chopped shallots**

**3 cloves garlic, minced**

**1 pound (455 g) sliced mushrooms**

**Salt and freshly ground black pepper to taste**

**1½ cups (270 g) Roasted Red Peppers, thinly sliced (see below)**

**2 cups (300 g) crumbled feta cheese**

① Preheat oven to 500°F (250°C, or gas mark 10). Roll each portion of dough into a 10-inch (25 cm) round and place on a baking sheet.

② Brush dough with vegetable shortening and bake in the oven for 5 minutes (this will keep it from getting soggy from the toppings). Let cool completely.

③ Meanwhile, heat olive oil in a large skillet over medium heat. Add shallots and cook, stirring often, for 5 to 6 minutes. Add garlic and mushrooms and cook, stirring often, for 5 minutes or until mushrooms are lightly browned. Season with salt and pepper. Remove from heat and spread in a single layer on a baking sheet to cool completely.

④ Top crust with mushroom mixture, roasted red peppers, and feta.

YIELD: 2 PIZZAS, OR 16 SERVINGS

## COOKING TIP: MAKE YOUR OWN ROASTED RED PEPPERS

Here's how to roast peppers: Preheat oven to 450°F (230°C, or gas mark 8). Cut stem end from peppers and remove seeds and membranes. Leave them whole or cut them in half. Place peppers on a roasting pan and roast for 10 to 15 minutes, turning every 5 minutes, until pepper skins are blistered and blackened. Remove from oven and place them in a large bowl covered with plastic wrap. Let them sweat for 20 minutes and then peel off most of the skins.

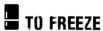 **TO FREEZE**

Wrap each pizza with freezer wrap or with a large sheet of plastic wrap and then aluminum foil.

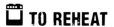 **TO REHEAT**

OVEN METHOD: Place a pizza stone in the oven and preheat oven to 425°F (220°C, or gas mark 7). Slide frozen pizza onto pizza stone and bake for 20 to 25 minutes or until crust is lightly browned and cheese is bubbling.

AMOUNT PER SERVING: Calories 217.94; Total Fat 7.95 g; Cholesterol 16.69 mg; Sodium 433.33 mg; Potassium 289.45 mg; Total Carbohydrates 30.09 g; Fiber 3.3 g; Sugar 2.16 g; Protein 8.3 g

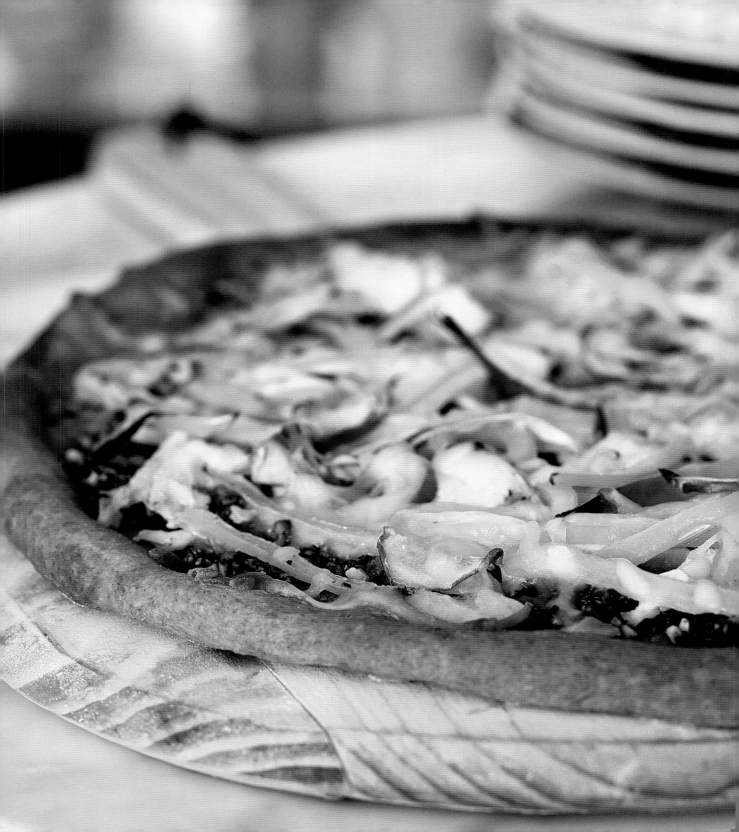

# BETTER-THAN-DELIVERY ROASTED CHICKEN PESTO PIZZA

A delectable change from tomato-sauced pizza, pesto is a perfect partner for roasted chicken breast, bell pepper, and cheese.

**2 portions fresh Whole-Grain Pizza Dough (page 138)**

**Vegetable shortening**

**1½ cups (290 g) Toasted Almond and Basil Pesto (page 169), and Hazelnut and Sun-Dried Tomato Pesto (page 167), or store-bought pesto**

**1 yellow bell pepper, seeded, halved, thinly sliced**

**½ small red onion, thinly sliced**

**2 cups (475 g) skinless shredded rotisserie chicken breast**

**3 cups (345 g) shredded mozzarella cheese**

① Preheat oven to 500°F (250°C, or gas mark 10). Roll each portion of dough into a 10-inch (25 cm) round and place on a baking sheet.

② Brush dough with vegetable shortening and bake in the oven for 5 minutes (this will keep it from getting soggy from the toppings). Let cool completely.

③ Spread pesto on dough and top with bell pepper, onion, chicken, and cheese.

YIELD: 2 PIZZAS, OR 16 SERVINGS

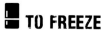 **TO FREEZE**

Wrap each pizza with freezer wrap or with a large sheet of plastic wrap and then aluminum foil.

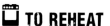 **TO REHEAT**

OVEN METHOD: Place a pizza stone in the oven and preheat oven to 425°F (220°C, or gas mark 7). Slide frozen pizza onto pizza stone and bake for 20 to 25 minutes or until crust is lightly browned and cheese is bubbling.

AMOUNT PER SERVING: Calories 333.32; Total Fat 15.71 g; Cholesterol 43.24 mg; Sodium 507 mg; Potassium 275.68 mg; Total Carbohydrates 27.31 g; Fiber 3.12 g; Sugar 1.38 g; Protein 21.43 g

# SOFT AND SEEDED OAT KNOTS

Fun for the kids and healthy for the family, these whole-grain goodies are perfect accompaniments for salads, soups, stews, and grilled meals.

¾ cup (175 ml) warm water

1 packet (2¼ teaspoons, or 9 g) active dry yeast

¼ cup (60 ml) warm milk

3 tablespoons (42 g) unsalted butter, softened at room temperature

1 tablespoon (13 g) granulated sugar

1 teaspoon salt

1½ cups (180 g) whole-wheat flour, divided

1 egg

1 cup (125 g) all-purpose flour

½ cup (45 g) oat flour

2 tablespoons (9 g) poppy seeds

2 tablespoons (18 g) sunflower seeds

2 tablespoons (16 g) sesame seeds

① Place ¼ cup (60 ml) warm water in the bowl of a standup mixer fitted with the paddle attachment. Sprinkle in yeast; stir until dissolved.

② Add remaining water, warm milk, butter, sugar, salt, and 1 cup (120 g) whole-wheat flour. Beat on medium speed until well-combined.

③ Add egg and ½ cup (60 g) whole-wheat flour, mixing until well-combined. Switch to the dough hook and add all-purpose flour, oat flour, and seeds. Knead dough on medium-high speed for 7 to 8 minutes or until dough is smooth and elastic. Dump onto a lightly floured surface and form into a ball.

④ Grease a large bowl and place dough in bowl, turning to coat with oil. Cover with a damp towel and set in a warm, draft-free place. Let dough rise for about 30 minutes.

⑤ Punch dough down and dump onto a lightly floured surface. Divide dough into 12 equal pieces and roll into an 8-inch (20 cm) rope. Tie each rope into a loose single knot.

YIELD: 12 KNOTS, OR 12 SERVINGS

## NUTRITION SPOTLIGHT: OAT FLOUR

Oat flour, made from ground oats, is a nutritious addition to baked goods. However, since it contains no gluten, it can't be used to replace wheat flour. You can find oat flour in the specialty baking aisle and at health food stores, or you can quickly make your own. To make oat flour, place rolled oats in a food processor or blender and grind into flour.

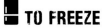 TO FREEZE

Place knots on a greased baking sheet and place in freezer just until solid. Transfer to a freezer bag, removing as much air as possible before sealing.

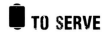 TO SERVE

Remove desired amount of knots from freezer and place them on a greased baking sheet. Cover with plastic and set in a warm, draft-free place. Let rise until doubled in size, about 1¼ hours.

OVEN METHOD: Bake at 350°F (180°C, or gas mark 4) for 15 minutes or until lightly browned and baked through.

AMOUNT PER SERVING: Calories 177.07; Total Fat 5.91 g; Cholesterol 25.56 mg; Sodium 213.88 mg; Potassium 117.96 mg; Total Carbohydrates 26.28 g; Fiber 1.82 g; Sugar 1.74 g; Protein 5.17 g

# QUICK TURKEY SAUSAGE AND BROCCOLI RABE CALZONES ✳

Calzones are tasty little pizza pouches that are a fun change from the classic flat pie. These calzones are given a healthy makeover with turkey sausage, a lean alternative to traditional pork sausage, super-veg broccoli rabe, and whole-grain pizza dough. For a change, substitute other vegetables for the broccoli rabe, add a swipe of marinara or pesto on the dough before filling, and try a medley of other cheeses.

........................................................................................

**2 tablespoons (28 ml) olive oil, plus more for brushing**

**1 small onion, diced**

**1 pound (455 g) hot or sweet turkey sausage**

**2 teaspoons dried oregano**

**2 teaspoons minced rosemary**

**2 cups (80 g) chopped, lightly steamed broccoli rabe**

**8 ounces (225 g) shredded mozzarella cheese**

**8 ounces (225 g) shredded provolone cheese**

**1 cup (80 g) shredded Parmesan cheese**

**2 portions fresh Whole-Grain Pizza Dough (page 138)**

① Heat oil in a large skillet over medium heat. Add onion and cook, stirring often, for 5 minutes. Add sausage, oregano, and rosemary and cook, stirring often, until sausage is lightly browned.

② Add broccoli rabe and cook, stirring often, for 3 to 4 minutes. Remove from heat and spread out onto a baking sheet to cool completely. In a medium bowl, mix together cheeses.

③ Place a baking stone in the oven and preheat oven to 500°F (250°C, or gas mark 10). Divide each portion of pizza dough into 3 or 4 pieces, rolling each piece into a ball. Roll each ball out into a flat round.

④ Top one half of each round with sausage mixture and cheese mixture, leaving a border. Fold dough over and tightly seal the edges. Brush with olive oil and slash the top of each calzone with a sharp knife.

⑤ Place calzones on pizza stone and bake for 7 to 8 minutes. They should be slightly underbaked. Transfer to wire racks to cool completely.

YIELD: 6 TO 8 CALZONES, OR 6 TO 8 SERVINGS

*Recipe continued on next page*

## NUTRITION SPOTLIGHT: BROCCOLI RABE

As part of the Brassica family, broccoli rabe is renowned for its cancer-fighting powers. It is an underappreciated nutritional star that is also a great source of vitamins A, C, and K as well as potassium, folic acid, iron, calcium, fiber, and flavonoids. Broccoli rabe, also called raab and rapini, hits its peak season in spring and can be quickly sautéed with olive oil and garlic for a simple super-healthy side dish.

AMOUNT PER SERVING: Calories 654.01; Total Fat 33.79 g; Sodium 1407.07 mg; Potassium 348.77 mg; Total Carbohydrates 54.21 g; Fiber 6.16 g; Sugar 3.14 g; Protein 35.71 g

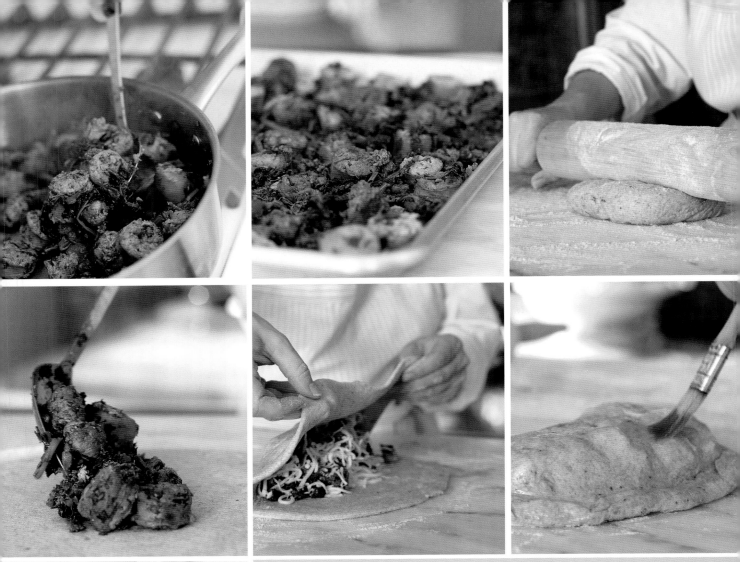

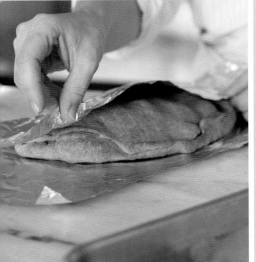

## TO FREEZE

Place calzones on a baking sheet and freeze until just solid. Wrap each calzone in aluminum foil.

## TO REHEAT

OVEN METHOD: Place pizza stone in oven and preheat oven to 350°F (180°C, or gas mark 4). Remove calzones from freezer and place on pizza stone while still in foil. Bake for 15 minutes. Open foil and continue to bake for 15 minutes or until crust is lightly browned and filling is hot.

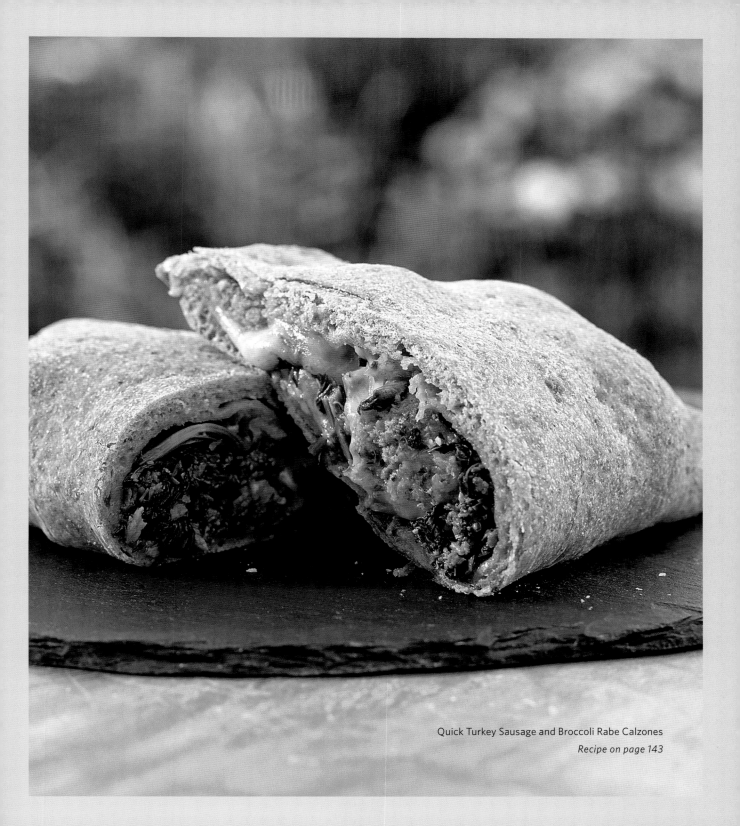

Quick Turkey Sausage and Broccoli Rabe Calzones

*Recipe on page 143*

# CHAPTER 8

# APPETIZERS
## BRING ON THE IMPROMPTU COCKTAIL PARTY

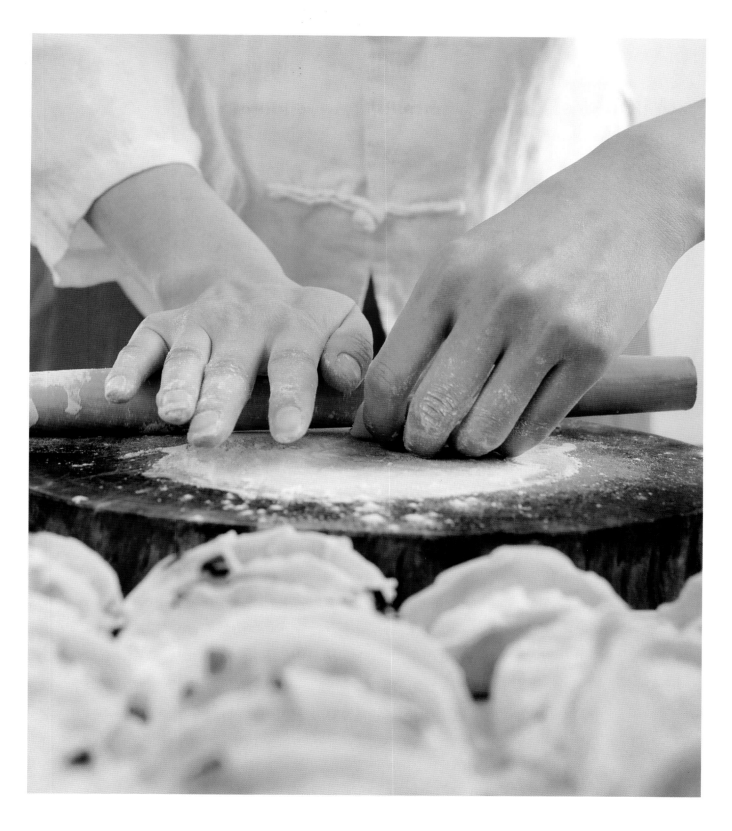

* Try

# MOUTHWATERING MINI CRAB CAKES

A tasty little nibble, these crab cakes are not only made with fiber-rich whole-wheat bread crumbs, they are baked in the oven instead of fried, saving you hundreds of appetizer calories. Serve with a low-fat tartar sauce or light wasabi mayonnaise.

**2 tablespoons (28 ml) olive oil**

**1 small onion, minced**

**1 carrot, minced**

**1 clove garlic, minced**

**1 pound (455 g) lump crab, picked over, finely chopped**

**⅔ cup (150 g) light mayonnaise made with olive oil**

**1 tablespoon (4 g) finely chopped fresh parsley**

**1 tablespoon (4 g) finely chopped fresh dill**

**1 tablespoon (3 g) finely chopped fresh chives**

**1 tablespoon (7 g) Old Bay Seasoning**

**2 tablespoons (22 g) Dijon mustard**

**5 cups (575 g) whole-wheat bread crumbs, divided**

**⅔ cup (83 g) all-purpose flour**

**4 eggs, beaten**

① Heat oil in a large skillet over medium heat. Add onion and carrot and cook, stirring often, for 5 minutes. Add garlic and cook, stirring, for 1 minute. Transfer to a large bowl.

② Add crab, mayonnaise, herbs, Old Bay, mustard, and 1 cup (115 g) bread crumbs. Form into 32 mini cakes.

③ Place flour in one shallow bowl, eggs in another shallow bowl, and remaining bread crumbs in a third shallow bowl. Dip crab cakes in flour, shaking off excess. Dip in eggs, allowing excess to drip off. Dip in bread crumbs to coat. Set on a greased baking sheet and refrigerate for 1 hour.

④ Preheat oven to 350°F (180°C, or gas mark 4). Spray crab cakes with cooking spray or brush with oil and bake for 20 to 25 minutes or until lightly browned. Let cool completely.

YIELD: 32 CRAB CAKES, OR 32 SERVINGS

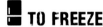

## TO FREEZE

Place crab cakes in freezer until firm. Transfer to a large freezer bag or freezer container.

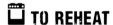

## TO REHEAT

MICROWAVE METHOD: Place desired number of crab cakes on a microwave-safe plate and heat on 50% power for 3 minutes or until heated through.

OVEN METHOD: Preheat oven to 375°F (190°C, or gas mark 5). Place crab cakes on a greased baking sheet and bake for 15 minutes or until heated through.

AMOUNT PER SERVING: Calories 221.7; Total Fat 14.64 g; Cholesterol 43 mg; Sodium 342.94 mg; Potassium 110.31 mg; Total Carbohydrates 15.68 g; Fiber 1.05 g; Sugar 1.45 g; Protein 6.37 g

# SIMPLY STUFFED CLAMS

Cooked seafood doesn't have an affinity for being frozen, but these stuffed clams certainly do. Best yet, they are quick and easy to make and can go straight from the freezer to the oven for those last-minute get-togethers when a nibble is a necessity. Pair it with your favorite Chardonnay. My picks are St. Francis Winery Behler Vineyard Chardonnay from Sonoma, California, and Cono Sur Vision Single Vineyard Chardonnay from the Casablanca Valley in Chile.

3 tablespoons (45 ml) olive oil

1 small onion, finely chopped

2 cloves garlic, minced

2 tablespoons (12 g) finely grated lemon zest

1 tablespoon (4 g) minced fresh parsley

2 tablespoons (6 g) minced fresh basil

Salt and freshly ground black pepper to taste

6 cans (6.5 ounces, or 185 g) minced clams, drained, liquid reserved

¾ cup (86 g) whole-wheat bread crumbs

Hot sauce to taste

36 clean clamshell halves

①  Heat oil in a medium skillet over medium heat. Add onion and cook, stirring often, until softened and lightly browned. Add garlic and lemon zest and cook, stirring, for 1 minute. Stir in parsley and basil and season with salt and pepper.

②  Remove from heat and add clams and bread crumbs, stirring to combine. Add just a few drops of hot sauce, taste, and decide if you want more. Add enough of the reserved clam liquid so that the mixture is very moist but holds together well. Spoon into the shells and let cool completely.

YIELD: 36 STUFFED CLAMS, OR 36 SERVINGS

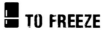 **TO FREEZE**

Place clams on a baking sheet and freeze until solid. Transfer to a freezer-safe container, layering with waxed paper.

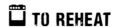 **TO REHEAT**

OVEN METHOD: Preheat oven to 350°F (180°C, or gas mark 4). Place frozen clams on baking sheet. Bake for 30 to 35 minutes.

AMOUNT PER SERVING:  Calories 47.86; Total Fat 1.57 g; Cholesterol 25.23 mg; Sodium 97.31 mg; Potassium 111.11 mg; Total Carbohydrates 1.91 g; Fiber 0.31 g; Sugar 0.18 g; Protein 6.25 g

# SLIM AND TRIM EMPAÑADAS

Tasty South American–style turnovers with spicy chicken sausage, black beans, and Manchego cheese are quick-to-the-table appetizers. Empañadas can be fried or baked after filling. This recipe forgoes deep frying and stays slim and trim from a bake in the oven. For a change, try different combinations of lower fat sausage, beans, and cheese.

FOR EMPAÑADAS:

**1 tablespoon (15 ml) olive oil**

**1 pound (455 g) spicy low-fat chicken sausage, casings removed, crumbled**

**½ cup (50 g) sliced scallions**

**2 cans (15 ounces, or 425 g, each) black beans, rinsed, drained**

**2 tablespoons (18 g) chipotle pepper in adobo sauce, finely chopped**

**3 portions Whole-Grain Pizza Dough (page 138)**

**3 cups (345 g) shredded Manchego cheese**

FOR SAUCE:

**2 tablespoons (28 ml) olive oil**

**½ cup (80 g) finely chopped onion**

**2 cloves garlic, crushed**

**2 cans (15 ounces, or 425 g, each) diced tomatoes**

**1 tablespoon (15 g) brown sugar**

**1 teaspoon dried oregano**

**½ teaspoon ground cumin**

**½ teaspoon ground coriander**

**Pinch of cayenne**

**Salt and freshly ground black pepper to taste**

① Preheat oven to 400°F (200°C, or gas mark 6).

② Heat oil in a large saucepan over medium heat. Cook sausage and onions, stirring often, until sausage is browned and onion in soft. Add black beans and chipotle and stir to combine. Remove from heat.

③ Line 2 baking sheets with parchment paper and spray with cooking spray. Set aside. On a lightly floured surface, roll 1 portion of dough into a 9 x 12-inch (23 x 30 cm) rectangle. Cut dough into 12 squares. Repeat with remaining 2 portions of dough.

④ Place a mound of sausage mixture on one half of each square, leaving a border, and top with cheese. Brush edges of squares with water and fold dough over to form triangles. Seal edges with tine of fork.

⑤ Place turnovers on prepared baking sheets. Brush turnovers with water. Bake in preheated over for 10 minutes. Transfer to wire racks to cool completely.

⑥ Meanwhile, in a medium saucepan over medium heat, heat olive oil for the sauce. Cook onion and garlic, stirring often, until onion is tender. Stir in tomatoes, sugar, oregano, cumin, coriander, and cayenne and bring to a boil.

⑦ Reduce heat and simmer, uncovered for 10 minutes or until most of the liquid has evaporated. Season with salt and pepper. Remove from heat and let cool.

YIELD: 36 TURNOVERS AND 3½ CUPS (858 G) SAUCE, OR 36 SERVINGS

## 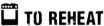 TO FREEZE

Place turnovers on a baking sheet and freeze until firm. Place in a 1-gallon (3.8 L) freezer bag, removing as much air as possible from bag before sealing. Transfer sauce to a freezer-safe container.

## TO REHEAT

Let turnovers and sauce thaw in the refrigerator overnight.

OVEN METHOD: Preheat oven to 425°F (220°C, or gas mark 7). Bake triangles on a baking sheet for 10 minutes or until golden brown. Reheat sauce over medium heat, stirring occasionally, for 5 to 6 minutes. If sauce is too thin, thicken it by whisking in 2 teaspoons cornstarch and 2 teaspoons water. Bring to a boil and stir. Serve turnovers with sauce. Sprinkle with extra Manchego cheese if desired.

AMOUNT PER SERVING: Calories 214.64; Total Fat 9.69 g; Cholesterol 2.09 mg; Sodium 216.73 mg; Potassium 199.54 mg; Total Carbohydrates 22.48 g; Fiber 3.73 g; Sugar 1.77 g; Protein 9.96 g

# LIGHT AND FLAKY SPANAKOPITA BITES

Inspired by the Greek spinach and cheese pie spanakopita, these tasty little bites are the perfect afternoon snack or accompaniment for a salad dinner on the nights you want something light and easy. Serve with Gazpacho with Vegetables Galore (page 82) or Garden Tomato Basil Soup (page 83).

**8 ounces (225 g) goat cheese, softened**

**1 tablespoon (6 g) minced lemon zest**

**3 tablespoons (45 ml) olive oil, divided**

**1 cup (160 g) finely chopped red onion**

**1 package (10 ounces, or 280 g) frozen spinach**

**1 tablespoon (2 g) fresh thyme**

**1 box (17.3 ounces, or 485 g) puff pastry, thawed**

① In a food processor, blend goat cheese, lemon zest, and 1 tablespoon (15 ml) olive oil.

② In a large skillet over medium heat, heat remaining oil and cook onion, stirring often, until onion is soft. Add spinach and cook, stirring occasionally, for 2 minutes. Add thyme and cook, stirring, for 1 minute. Remove from heat and allow to cool completely.

③ Add spinach mixture to cheese mixture and pulse to combine.

④ Roll puff pastry into two 12-inch (30 cm) squares. Cut each square into sixteen 3-inch (7.5 cm) squares. Brush edges of puff pastry with water. Place a dollop of spinach-cheese mixture on the center of each square and fold to form triangles, pressing the edges to seal.

YIELD: 32 BITES, OR 32 SERVINGS

*Recipe continued on next page*

---

### NUTRITION SPOTLIGHT: GIVE GOAT CHEESE A GO

If cheese made from cow milk causes you digestive distress, cheese derived from goat milk may be your ticket to a tummy-happy dairy intake. Believe it or not, goat milk bears similar characteristics to human milk, making goat milk and goat cheese easier to digest, especially for people who are lactose sensitive or intolerant. Goat cheese is also lower in fat, calories, and cholesterol than cow-derived cheese and is a delicious source of bone-building calcium.

---

AMOUNT PER SERVING: Calories 119.61; Total Fat 8.7 g; Cholesterol 3.26 mg; Sodium 92.89 mg; Potassium 38.66 mg; Total Carbohydrates 7.83 g; Fiber 0.67 g; Sugar 0.23 g; Protein 2.84 g

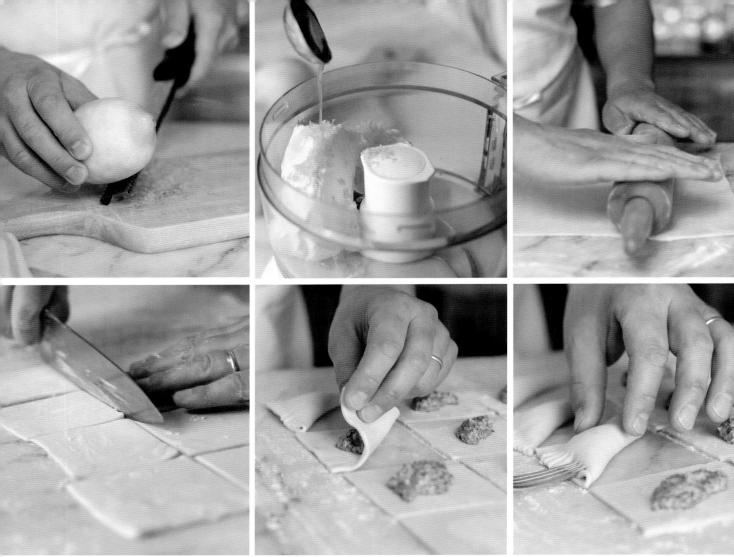

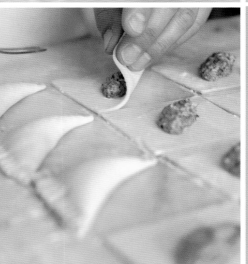

## TO FREEZE

Arrange triangles on a baking sheet and freeze until firm. Place in a 1 gallon-size (3.8 L) freezer bag, removing as much air as possible from bag before sealing

## TO REHEAT

Let triangles thaw in the refrigerator overnight. Preheat oven to 425°F (220°C, or gas mark 7). Place triangles on a baking sheet and bake for 15 minutes or until puff pastry is golden brown. Let cool for 10 minutes before serving.

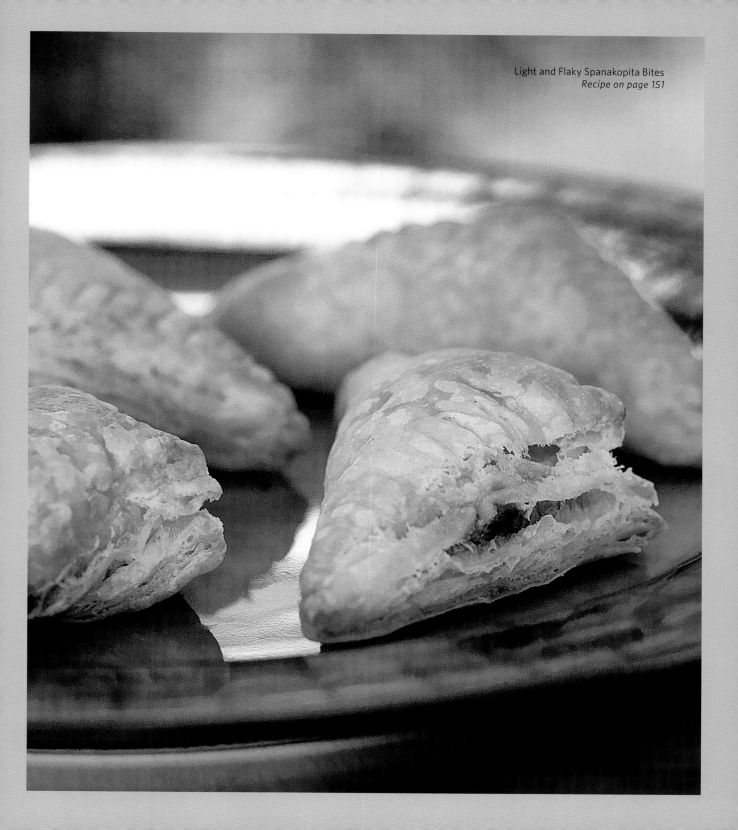

Light and Flaky Spanakopita Bites
*Recipe on page 151*

# TASTY TURKEY MEATBALLS

Meatballs are a must-serve for easy entertaining. Hearty little mouthfuls of curry-flavored ground turkey give these meatballs a tasty edge—they are not only a welcome change from the usual beef meatball, they are lower in fat and offer the heart-healthy benefit of curry powder.

**1½ pounds (680 g) lean ground turkey breast**

**1 cup (160 g) finely chopped red onion**

**1 egg**

**¼ cup (60 ml) milk**

**⅓ cup (38 g) dry whole-wheat bread crumbs or Whole-Grain Bread Crumbs (page 175)**

**1 teaspoon salt**

**Freshly ground black pepper to taste**

**1 tablespoon (15 g) brown sugar**

**1 tablespoon (6 g) curry powder**

**3 tablespoons (3 g) finely chopped fresh cilantro**

① Preheat oven to 400°F (200°C, or gas mark 6). Mix all ingredients in a large bowl. Shape into 36 meatballs.

② Place on a large greased rimmed baking sheet and spray with cooking spray. Bake for 20 minutes or until meatballs are browned and cooked through. Let cool completely.

YIELD: 36 MEATBALLS, OR 36 SERVINGS

## NUTRITION SPOTLIGHT: CURRY POWDER

Curry powder, that distinctive flavored, bright-colored yellow spice blend, is one of the most delicious ways to derail disease. Curry powder gets its super-spice status from turmeric, a peppery, warm, and astringent spice that gives curry flavor and hue. Turmeric has long been used as an anti-inflammatory in ancient Chinese medicine, but recent research suggests that curcumin, the yellow-orange pigment in this super-spice, has the same anti-inflammatory power as prescription and over-the-counter medicines.

 **TO FREEZE**

Place meatballs on a rimmed baking sheet and freeze until firm. Place in a large freezer bag, removing as much air as possible before sealing.

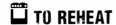 **TO REHEAT**

STOVETOP METHOD: Heat 2 tablespoons (28 ml) oil in a large skillet over medium heat. Add meatballs, cooking in batches if necessary, and cook, stirring occasionally, for 7 minutes or until meatballs are heated through.

OVEN METHOD: Preheat oven to 350°F (180°C, or gas mark 4) and place meatballs on a greased rimmed baking sheet. Bake, turning occasionally, for 25 to 30 minutes or until heated through.

AMOUNT PER SERVING: Calories 30.44; Total Fat 0.57 g; Cholesterol 14.17 mg; Sodium 267.91 mg; Potassium 67.5 mg; Total Carbohydrates 2.51 g; Fiber 0.27 g; Sugar 1.24 g; Protein 3.68 g

# QUICK LOW-CARB MINI QUICHE ✳ Int

Crustless quiche is not only easier to make, it's lower in fat and carbs. These cheesy custard bites are also quick to reheat. For a tasty change, substitute other veggies or cheese you have on hand. Make a few different batches and serve an assortment of mini quiche at your next get-together.

**1½ cups (340 g) low-fat cottage cheese**

**3 eggs (or ¾ cup [170 g] Egg Beaters to further reduce fat)**

**3 tablespoons (23 g) baking mix**

**1 cup (180 g) finely chopped Roasted Red Peppers (page 139)**

**½ cup (50 g) finely chopped scallions (white and green parts)**

**2 cups (240 g) shredded Gouda cheese**

**2 tablespoons (6 g) finely chopped fresh basil**

**Salt and freshly ground black pepper to taste**

① Preheat oven to 350°F (180°C, or gas mark 4) and grease two 24-cup mini-muffin pans.

② Place cottage cheese in a food processor and blend until smooth. In a large bowl, whisk together eggs and baking mix. Stir in peppers, scallions, Gouda, and basil. Season with salt and pepper.

③ Bake for 15 minutes or until quiche are puffed and golden. Remove from oven and invert onto wire racks to cool completely.

YIELD: 48 MINI QUICHE, OR 48 SERVINGS

## NUTRITION TIP: GO EASY ON THE LOW-CARB LIFESTYLE

You can certainly lose weight by cutting out high-carb foods—it usually means you are also consuming fewer calories—but eschewing breads, rice, pasta, and other carb-rich foods for long periods of time is not only challenging, it isn't a sensible, balanced approach to eating. Instead of swearing off all carbs, simply comprise your carbohydrate choices of whole grains, fruits and vegetables, and steer clear of the refined flour and packaged foods.

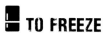 ## TO FREEZE

INDIVIDUAL SERVINGS: Place quiche on a large baking sheet and freeze until solid. Place in a large freezer bag, removing as much air as possible before sealing.

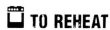 ## TO REHEAT

OVEN METHOD: Preheat oven to 350°F (180°C, or gas mark 4). Place quiche on a baking sheet and bake for 12 to 15 minutes or until heated through. Serve warm or at room temperature.

AMOUNT PER SERVING: Calories 31.04; Total Fat 1.79 g; Cholesterol 18.85 mg; Sodium 82.23 mg; Potassium 25.77 mg; Total Carbohydrates 1.2 g; Fiber 0.14 g; Sugar 0.37 g; Protein 2.56 g

# HEALTHY JALAPEÑO POPPERS

Jalapeños stuffed with meat and cheese are a fiery finger food that effortlessly evoke groans of satisfaction. For a change, swap out the turkey sausage with shrimp, taking care not to overcook it.

......................................................

**24 red or green jalapeño peppers, stem end trimmed, seeded**

**1 tablespoon (15 ml) olive oil**

**4 ounces (115 g) hot Italian turkey sausage, casing removed, crumbled**

**¼ cup (40 g) finely chopped onion**

**1 teaspoon dried oregano**

**1 teaspoon chili powder**

**½ teaspoon ground coriander**

**Salt and freshly ground black pepper**

**4 ounces (115 g) goat cheese, softened at room temperature**

**4 ounces (115 g) Neufchâtel cheese, softened at room temperature**

**¾ cup (175 ml) milk**

**1 egg, beaten**

**1 cup (125 g) all-purpose flour**

**1½ cups (175 g) dry whole-wheat bread crumbs**

① Bring a large pot of water to a boil over high heat. Add jalapeños and blanch for 2 to 3 minutes. Transfer to paper towels to drain. Pat dry and make sure water is drained out of peppers.

② Heat oil in a medium skillet over medium-high heat. Cook turkey sausage and onion, stirring often, until onion is softened and turkey sausage is browned. Season with oregano, chili powder, coriander, and salt and pepper. Set aside to cool.

③ In a food processor, combine goat cheese and Neufchâtel and blend until smooth. Add sausage mixture and pulse to combine. Spoon or pipe cheese mixture into jalapeños.

④ In a shallow dish, whisk together milk and egg. In a second shallow dish, combine flour and a pinch of salt and pepper. Place bread crumbs in a third shallow dish.

⑤ Dip jalapeños in milk mixture, letting excess drain off. Dip in flour mixture and set on a wire rack until coating is dry. Dip jalapeños again in milk mixture and then roll in bread crumbs, repeating if necessary. Set on wire racks again to dry.

YIELD: 24 POPPERS, OR 24 SERVINGS

## COOKING TIP: KEEP THE HEAT IN THE JALAPEÑO

Handling the occasional jalapeño for salsa or another spicy dish is usually a pain-free endeavor, as long as you don't rub your eyes. However, trimming and seeding two dozen peppers can irritate your skin. To prevent the heat-emitting oil, capsicum, from burning your fingers, put on a pair of dishwashing gloves before you start prepping jalapeños.

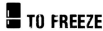

## TO FREEZE

Place poppers on a baking sheet and freeze until solid. Transfer to a freezer container, placing a piece of waxed paper in between layers.

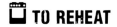

## TO REHEAT

OVEN METHOD: Preheat oven to 350°F (180°C, or gas mark 4). Place poppers on a baking sheet and bake for 25 minutes or until heated through and lightly browned.

AMOUNT PER SERVING: Calories 68.96; Total Fat 3.97 g; Cholesterol 18.37 mg; Sodium 72.77 mg; Potassium 51.09 mg; Total Carbohydrates 5.4 g; Fiber 0.65 g; Sugar 0.64 g; Protein 3.1 g

# BAKED VEGGIE AND SHRIMP EGG ROLLS

A medley of veggies and tender shrimp tucked in a wrap and baked to warm perfection make these egg rolls a healthy alternative to deep-fried varieties.

**3 tablespoons (45 ml) peanut oil**

**1 bunch scallions, trimmed, finely chopped (white and green parts)**

**1 small head napa cabbage, thinly sliced crosswise, finely chopped**

**3 carrots, shredded**

**1 pound (455 g) salad shrimp, finely chopped**

**1 can (8 ounces, or 225 g) water chestnuts, drained, finely chopped**

**½ pound (225 g) fresh bean sprouts, finely chopped**

**4 cloves garlic, minced**

**2 tablespoons (32 g) smooth peanut butter**

**1 tablespoon (15 ml) tamari**

**1 tablespoon (15 ml) sesame oil**

**32 egg roll wrappers**

① Heat oil in a large wok over medium-high heat. Add scallions, cabbage, and carrots and stir-fry until tender. Add shrimp, water chestnuts, bean sprouts, and garlic and stir-fry for 1 minute.

② In a small bowl, whisk together peanut butter, tamari, and sesame oil. Pour into wok and toss with vegetable mixture to coat. Remove from heat and spread out on a rimmed baking sheet to cool completely.

③ Mound filling onto the center of each egg roll wrapper, fold top and bottom edges over, and then wrap into a roll. Set on a clean baking sheet.

YIELD: 32 EGG ROLLS, OR 32 SERVINGS

*Recipe continued on next page*

AMOUNT PER SERVING: Calories 138.97; Total Fat 2.93 g; Cholesterol 38.71 mg; Sodium 354.15 mg; Potassium 99.91 mg; Total Carbohydrates 21.12 g; Fiber 1.25 g; Sugar 1 g; Protein 6.74 g

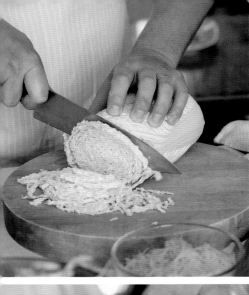

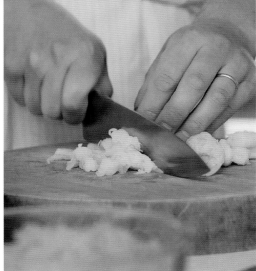

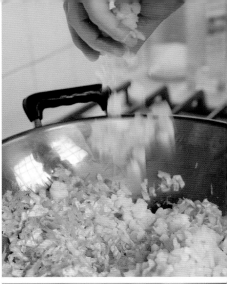

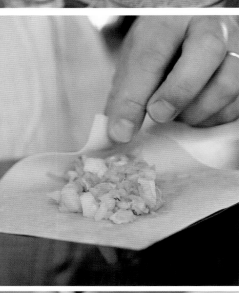

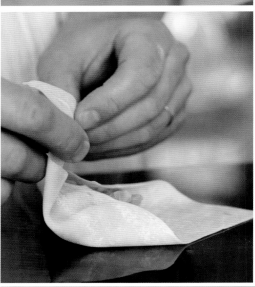

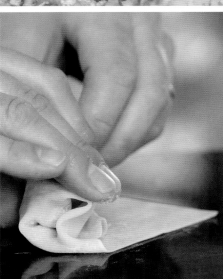

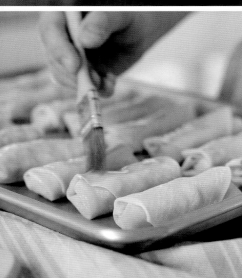

## ❄ TO FREEZE

Set baking sheet in freezer until egg rolls are solid. Transfer to a large freezer bag or freezer-safe container.

## ⊡ TO REHEAT

Thaw egg rolls in the refrigerator overnight.

OVEN METHOD: Preheat oven to 375°F (190°C, or gas mark 5). Place egg rolls on a greased baking sheet and generously spray with cooking spray or brush with canola oil. Bake for 15 to 20 minutes or until heated through and lightly browned.

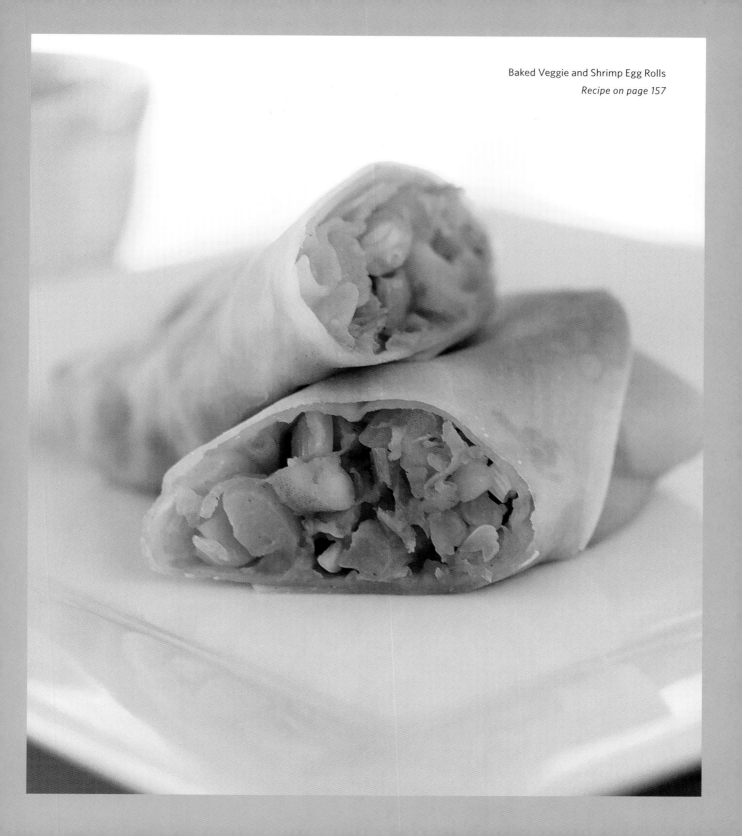

Baked Veggie and Shrimp Egg Rolls
*Recipe on page 157*

# BAKE-AHEAD FIG AND BRIE TARTLETS

Figs and brie are a delectable pair, but fresh figs have a short season and running off to the store for a round of brie isn't necessarily convenient. Fix and freeze a batch or two of these savory sweet tartlets, and you can have a divine bite of figs and cheese in under 15 minutes. You can also use Spicy Blackberry Freezer Jam (page 172) for a change or if fig preserves aren't available.

**1 package (15 ounces, or 425 g) refrigerated pie crusts**

**1 round (8 ounces, or 225 g) brie, rind removed, room temperature**

**½ cup (55 g) chopped candied pecans**

**1 cup (320 g) fig preserves**

**1 scallion, minced (green and white parts)**

**1½ teaspoons balsamic vinegar**

**1 teaspoon minced fresh rosemary**

**Salt and freshly ground black pepper to taste**

① Preheat oven to 425°F (220°C, or gas mark 7).

② Unroll pie crust on a flat surface. Cut into 48 rounds using a 2-inch (5 cm) round cutter. Press rounds into bottoms of prepared mini-muffin pans, pressing dough against the sides of each cup. Prick bottom of dough with a fork.

③ Bake crusts for 5 minutes. Cool on a wire rack. Reduce oven temperature to 300°F (150°C, or gas mark 2).

④ Place brie in a food processor and blend until smooth. Spoon or pipe brie into pastry cups. Sprinkle with pecans, lightly pressing them down into brie. Bake for 4 minutes or until brie just melts. Transfer to wire rack.

⑤ In a bowl, whisk together fig preserves, scallion, balsamic, and rosemary. Season with salt and pepper. Place a spoonful of fig preserves mixture on each brie cup. Let cups cool completely.

YIELD: 48 TARTLETS, OR 48 SERVINGS

 **TO FREEZE**

Place tartlets on a baking sheet and freeze until solid. Transfer to a freezer container with a sheet of waxed paper in between each layer. You can also freeze tartlets in muffin pans covered tightly with freezer wrap.

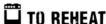 **TO REHEAT**

OVEN METHOD: Preheat oven to 375°F (190°C, or gas mark 5). Place frozen tartlets on a baking sheet and bake for 10 to 12 minutes or until heated through.

Amount Per Serving: Calories 88.03; Total Fat 4.93 g; Cholesterol 4.73 mg; Sodium 92.59 mg; Potassium 23.25 mg; Total Carbohydrates 9.39 g; Fiber 0.26 g; Sugar 3.83 g; Protein 1.49 g

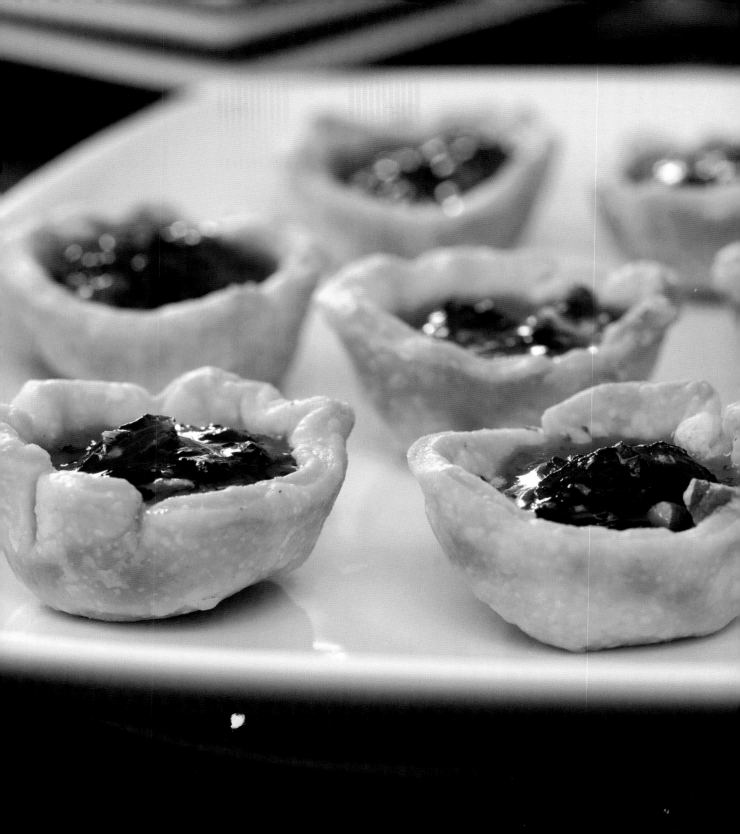

# CHAPTER 9

# SAUCES, CONDIMENTS, AND OTHER STAPLES
## COMPLEMENTING YOUR FREEZER-FRIENDLY MEALS

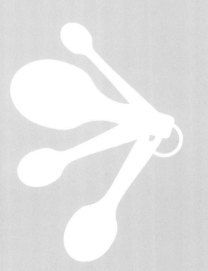

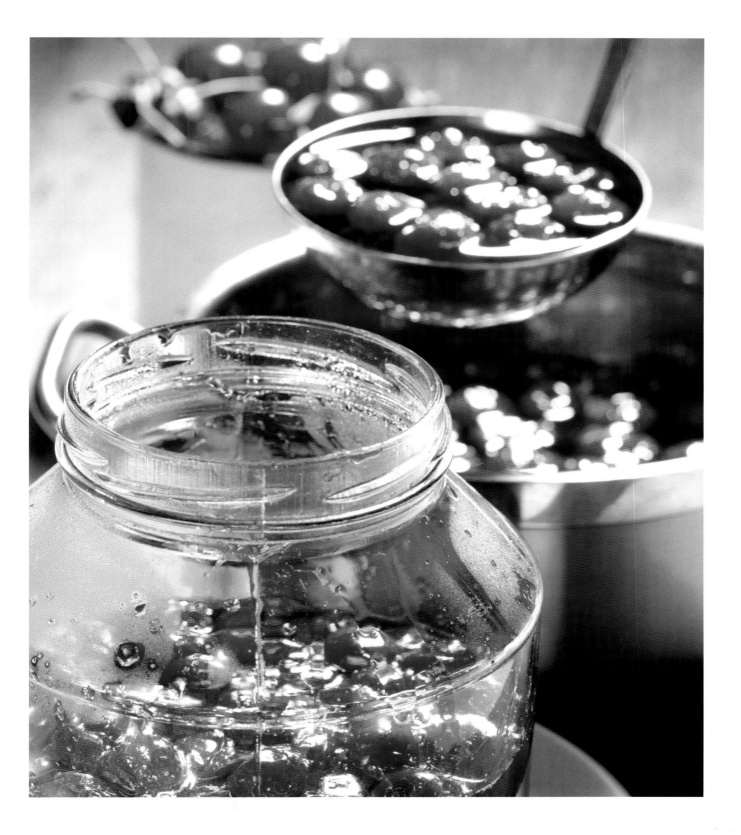

# SUPER-FAST EVERYDAY PEANUT SAUCE

Creamy, spicy, and nutty, toss this sassy sauce with pasta, drizzle it over vegetables, or use it as a dipping sauce for Party-Perfect Pork and Veggie Dumplings (page 54).

........................................................................................................................

**1½ cups (390 g) smooth peanut butter**

**1 cup (235 ml) light coconut milk**

**3 tablespoons (45 ml) tamari**

**2 tablespoons (28 ml) toasted sesame oil**

**2 tablespoons (2 ml) fish sauce**

**3 tablespoons (24 g) grated fresh ginger**

**2 cloves garlic, pressed**

**1½ teaspoons red pepper flakes**

**3 tablespoons (3 g) finely chopped fresh cilantro**

**Salt to taste**

**Ground white pepper to taste**

① In the bowl of a food processor, combine all ingredients and blend until smooth.

YIELD: ABOUT 3 CUPS (675 G), OR 12 SERVINGS

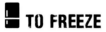 **TO FREEZE**

Place sauce in a freezer bag or freezer container.

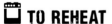 **TO REHEAT**

Let sauce thaw in refrigerator overnight.

STOVETOP METHOD: **Place sauce in a saucepan over medium heat and cook, stirring often, until it comes to a simmer. Reduce heat to low and stir until heated through.**

> AMOUNT PER SERVING: Calories 254.46; Total Fat 22.78 g; Cholesterol 0 mg; Sodium 422.98 mg; Potassium 276.48 mg; Total Carbohydrates 7.70 g; Fiber 2.04 g; Sugar 3.12 g; Protein 9.12 g

# EGGPLANT AND ROASTED RED PEPPER SPREAD

The popularity of the Mediterranean diet has created a surge of Mediterranean products, including sauces and other condiments. You can make your own Mediterranean-inspired sauces for a fraction of the cost (and calories) of store-bought products. This thick, flavorful eggplant sauce is a sensational bruschetta spread, pasta sauce, and topping for meats, poultry, and seafood.

**2 eggplants (1 pound, or 455 g, each), halved lengthwise**

**3 tablespoons (45 ml) olive oil, divided**

**1 large red onion, finely chopped**

**5 cloves garlic, minced**

**2 cups (360 g) roasted red peppers packed in water, diced**

**2 cups (220 g) sun-dried tomatoes packed in olive oil, drained, chopped**

**Grated zest and juice of 1 large lemon**

**½ cup (120 ml) red wine**

**½ cup (120 ml) water**

**½ cup (20 g) finely chopped fresh basil**

① Preheat the oven to 350°F (180°C, or gas mark 4).

② Brush eggplant with 1 tablespoon (15 ml) olive oil and place halves, cut-side down, in a baking pan. Bake for 1 hour or until tender. Let cool and then scoop out flesh. Discard the skin and then chop.

③ Heat remaining olive oil in a Dutch oven over medium heat. Add onion and cook, stirring often, for 8 minutes or until softened. Add garlic and cook, stirring, for 1 minute.

④ Add peppers, sun-dried tomatoes, lemon zest and juice, wine, and water, stirring to combine. Stir in eggplant, tossing to combine, and bring to a low boil. Lower heat to low and simmer, stirring occasionally, for 10 to 15 minutes or until mixture thickens slightly. Stir in basil. Remove from heat and allow to cool completely.

YIELD: 12 CUPS (2.9 KG), OR 24 SERVINGS

 **TO FREEZE**

Transfer sauce to one or two 1-gallon (3.8 L) freezer bags and lay flat in a casserole dish. Freeze until solid and then remove casserole dish.

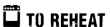 **TO REHEAT**

Let sauce thaw in the refrigerator overnight.

MICROWAVE METHOD: Pour sauce into a microwave-safe container. Cover loosely and reheat on 60% power for 2 minutes for small servings and up to 5 minutes for larger portions.

STOVETOP METHOD: Pour sauce into a saucepan over medium-high heat and cook, stirring occasionally, for 10 minutes or until heated through.

AMOUNT PER SERVING: Calories 54.83; Total Fat 3.12 g; Cholesterol 0 mg; Sodium 26.17 mg; Potassium 265.36 mg; Total Carbohydrates 6.26 g; Fiber 2.38 g; Sugar 0.94 g; Protein 1.12 g

# MUST-MAKE MARINARA SAUCE

Store-bought marinara is a convenient grab, but often it is laden with sugar and lacks the depth of flavor a sauce simmered on the stove with your family's favorite ingredients. This sauce can be used for the usual pasta bake, but it can also layer lasagna, fill calzones, and top pizzas. For a vegetarian version, omit the sausage and add tempeh or kidney beans.

**3 tablespoons (45 ml) olive oil**

**2 pounds (900 g) Italian turkey sausage, casings removed, crumbled**

**2 onions, chopped**

**1 large zucchini, finely chopped**

**2 tablespoons (4 g) minced fresh rosemary**

**2 teaspoons dried oregano**

**5 cloves garlic, minced**

**1 cup (235 ml) red wine**

**2 tablespoons (28 ml) balsamic vinegar**

**3 jars (25 ounces, or 700 g, each) commercial low-sugar marinara sauce**

**2 cans (28 ounces, or 785 g, each) fire-roasted diced tomatoes, or 7 cups (1.3 kg) Fire-Roasted Tomatoes (page 39)**

**1 cup (175 g) finely chopped dried plums**

**Salt and freshly ground black pepper to taste**

① Heat oil in a large stockpot over medium heat. Brown sausage and transfer with a slotted spoon to a large plate.

② Add onions and zucchini. Cook, stirring often, until onions are softened. Add rosemary, oregano, and garlic. Cook, stirring often, until garlic is fragrant. Stir in red wine and vinegar, scraping the bottom of the pan to remove browned bits.

③ Add marinara sauce, diced tomatoes, dried plums, and sausage. Increase heat to medium-high and bring to a boil. Reduce heat to medium-low and simmer, uncovered, for 30 minutes. Taste and season with salt and pepper. Continue to simmer for 15 to 20 minutes. Remove from heat and allow to cool.

YIELD: 18 CUPS (4.4 KG), OR 36 SERVING

## NUTRITION SPOTLIGHT: DRIED PLUMS (AKA PRUNES)

Many commercial tomato sauces are made with a generous addition of sugar. Instead of turning to granulated sugar to balance the flavor of your marinaras, add dried plums. Not only are dried plums naturally sweet, they are loaded with antioxidants (something sugar can't claim) and give sauces a thicker texture. You don't have to stop with tomato sauce; add dried plums to your grain dishes, stir them into your oatmeal or cold cereal, and substitute them (chopped) for raisins in other recipes.

 **TO FREEZE**

Transfer sauce to 1-gallon (3.8 L) freezer bags. Lay bags in a baking dish and freeze. Remove baking dish and stack bags in freezer.

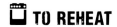 **TO REHEAT**

Thaw in the refrigerator overnight.

STOVETOP METHOD: Reheat in a saucepan over medium heat.

AMOUNT PER SERVING: Calories 170.56; Total Fat 7.7 g; Cholesterol 21.31 mg; Sodium 413.69 mg; Potassium 486.72 mg; Total Carbohydrates 18.25 g; Fiber 3.85 g; Sugar 10.25 g; Protein 5.58 g

*Adapt — exper. w/ oil & cutting it down.*

# HAZELNUT AND SUN-DRIED TOMATO PESTO

An inventive variation on traditional pesto, this recipe showcases sun-dried tomatoes and the earthy flavor of hazelnuts. Delicious with pasta and as a spread for burgers, try it as a wholesome dip for chicken fingers or sweet potato fries.

⅓ **cup (45 g) hazelnuts**

2 cups (48 g) firmly packed fresh
basil leaves

½ cup (55 g) sun-dried tomatoes
in olive oil, drained

5 cloves garlic

¼ cup (25 g) freshly grated
Parmesan cheese

¼ cup (25 g) freshly grated
pecorino Romano cheese

Zest and juice of 1 lemon

¾ cup (175 ml) extra-virgin olive oil

Salt and freshly ground black
pepper

① Place hazelnuts, basil, sun-dried tomatoes, garlic, cheeses, and lemon zest and juice in a food processor. Blend until finely chopped.

② With motor running, drizzle in olive oil until a smooth sauce forms. Season with salt and pepper.

YIELD: 2½ CUPS (650 G), OR 10 SERVINGS

 **TO FREEZE**

Transfer to a 1-quart (950 ml) freezer bag, removing as much air as possible before sealing. For small portions, such as garnish for soup or whisking into a dressing, you can also freeze in ice cube trays until solid and then transfer cubes to a 1-quart (950 ml) freezer bag.

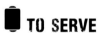 **TO SERVE**

Place freezer bag in the refrigerator overnight to thaw. If using cubes, place desired amount in a small bowl and thaw in the refrigerator.

OVEN METHOD: For warm dishes or to use as a sauce, you can heat on low.

AMOUNT PER SERVING: Calories 210.19; Total Fat 21.21 g; Cholesterol 4.8 mg; Sodium 83.99 mg; Potassium 167.12 mg; Total Carbohydrates 4.13 g; Fiber 1.41 g; Sugar 0.31 g; Protein 3.17 g

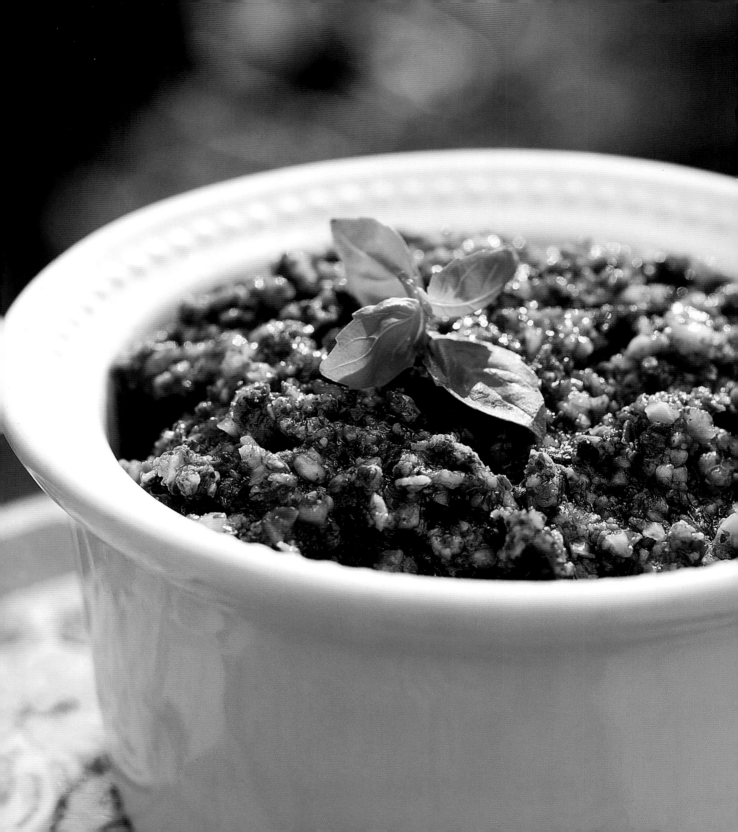

# TOASTED ALMOND AND BASIL PESTO

*Experiment w/ cutting down oil.*

Pesto is not only a versatile Italian-inspired sauce, it is chock-full of nutrient-dense ingredients. Traditionally made with pine nuts, this recipe features almonds toasted to tasty perfection. Pesto can be tossed with pasta, layered in lasagna, used as a wrap or sandwich spread, added to omelets, and whisked into a vinaigrette.

½ cup (73 g) raw almonds

2 cups (48 g) firmly packed fresh basil leaves

4 cloves garlic

½ cup (50 g) freshly grated Parmesan cheese

1 tablespoon (6 g) grated lemon zest

2 tablespoons (28 ml) fresh lemon juice

½ cup (120 ml) extra-virgin olive oil

Salt and freshly ground black pepper to taste

① Preheat oven to 350°F (180°C, or gas mark 4). Spread nuts in a single layer on a baking sheet. Toast in the oven for 6 minutes or until nuts are golden and fragrant. Set aside to cool slightly.

② When nuts are cool to the touch, transfer to the food processor. Add basil, garlic, cheese, lemon zest, and lemon juice. Pulse until finely chopped.

③ With the motor running, drizzle in olive oil and blend until combined. Season with salt and pepper.

YIELD: 2 CUPS (520 G), OR 8 SERVINGS

 **TO FREEZE**

Transfer to a 1-quart (950 ml) freezer bag, removing as much air as possible before sealing. For small portions, such as garnish for soup or whisking into a dressing, you can also freeze in ice cube trays until solid and then transfer cubes to a 1-quart (950 ml) freezer bag.

 **TO SERVE**

Place freezer bag in the refrigerator overnight to thaw. If using cubes, place desired amount in a small bowl and thaw in the refrigerator.

STOVETOP METHOD: For warm dishes or to use as a sauce, you can heat on low.

AMOUNT PER SERVING: Calories 205.68; Total Fat 20.05 g; Cholesterol 5.5 mg; Sodium 96.56 mg; Potassium 106.1 mg; Total Carbohydrates 3.36 g; Fiber 1.36 g; Sugar 0.57 g; Protein 4.7 g

# FIVE-WAYS FRESH HERB SPREAD

Thicker than a pesto and sans cheese, this herb paste can become an intensely flavored spread for bread, tossed with warm pasta or rice for a quick side dish, stirred into mashed potatoes, or thinned down to drizzle on vegetables, poultry, or fish. You can even swirl it into eggs for a garden-fresh omelet.

½ cup (30 g) fresh flat-leaf parsley

½ cup (12 g) fresh basil leaves

3 tablespoons (5 g) fresh rosemary

Grated zest and juice of 1 small orange

2 cloves garlic, chopped

1 cup (100 g) chopped scallions

⅓ cup (80 ml) extra-virgin olive oil

Salt and freshly ground black pepper to taste

 Combine parsley, basil, rosemary, orange zest and juice, garlic, and scallions in a food processor and pulse to coarsely chop.

 With machine running, slowly pour in oil, blending until a paste forms. Season with salt and pepper.

YIELD: 2¼ CUPS (585 G), OR 8 SERVINGS

## ▐ TO FREEZE

Transfer to a 1-quart (950 ml) freezer bag, removing as much air as possible before sealing. For small portions, such as garnish for soup or whisking into a dressing, you can also freeze in ice cube trays until solid and then transfer cubes to a 1-quart (950 ml) freezer bag.

## ▐ TO SERVE

Place freezer bag in the refrigerator overnight to thaw. If using cubes, place desired amount in a small bowl and thaw in the refrigerator.

STOVETOP METHOD: For warm dishes or to use as a sauce, you can heat on low.

AMOUNT PER SERVING:  Calories 98.93; Total Fat 9.07 g; Cholesterol 0 mg; Sodium 5.04 mg; Potassium 107.03 mg; Total Carbohydrates 4.66 g; Fiber 1.48 g; Sugar 0.34 g; Protein 0.73 g

# HOT AND HEALTHY SPICE BLEND

Give your next chili or tortilla soup some heat with this spicy blend. You can also blend this with mayonnaise or cream cheese for a hot gourmet spread for wraps and sandwiches.

⅓ cup (43 g) chili powder

3 tablespoons (21 g) ground cumin

2 tablespoons (3.4 g) dried onion flakes

1 tablespoon (3 g) dried oregano

1 tablespoon (6 g) ground coriander

1 tablespoon (9 g) garlic powder

½ teaspoon ground cinnamon

½ teaspoon chipotle powder

1 teaspoon salt

Freshly ground black pepper to taste

① In a bowl, combine all ingredients.

YIELD: ¾ CUP (32 G)
SERVINGS: 20 (0.3 OUNCE)

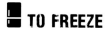 **TO FREEZE**

Place in a freezer bag or freezer-safe container.

 **TO USE**

Portion out the amount needed.

AMOUNT PER YIELD:  Calories 13.55; Total Fat 0.66 g; Cholesterol 0 mg; Sodium 133.39 mg; Potassium 78.98 mg; Total Carbohydrates 2.3 g; Fiber 0.99 g; Sugar 0.36 g; Protein 0.6 g

# SPICY BLACKBERRY FREEZER JAM

Stock up on these juicy dark-hued berries at your farmers' market when they are at their peak during the summer season. This spicy blackberry jam can be slathered on your breakfast treats, swirled into baked goods, or even used as a sweet sauce for chicken, pork, or salmon. It is especially delish on Quick and Easy English Muffin Toaster Waffles (page 180) or Oat-Rageous Cinnamon Brown Sugar Waffles (page 181).

**2 packages (1.59 ounces, or 45 g, each) freezer jam fruit pectin**

**3 cups (600 g) granulated sugar**

**8 cups (1.2 kg) crushed blackberries**

**1 teaspoon ground cinnamon**

**1 teaspoon freshly ground nutmeg**

**½ teaspoon ground cardamom**

**Juice and grated zest of 1 small lemon**

**10 plastic freezer jars (8 ounces, or 235 g)**

① In a large bowl, stir together pectin and sugar.

② Add blackberries, cinnamon, nutmeg, cardamom, lemon juice, and lemon zest to sugar and stir until well-combined, further crushing blackberries.

③ Using a funnel, spoon jam into freezer jars to fill line. Twist on lids. Let stand for 30 minutes or until thickened.

YIELD: TEN 8-OUNCE (227 G) JARS
(SERVINGS SIZE IS 1 TABLESPOON, OR 20 G)

## COOKING TIP: MAKE FAST AND BUDGET-FRIENDLY FREEZER JAM

Freezer jam is a super-easy way to preserve fruit because it doesn't require boiling water or extra pots and pans on the stove. It is also economical because you won't waste a single fruit and jars of homemade freezer jam are cheaper than store-bought jams. Make a variety of freezer jams and the next slather of fruit goodness is as close as your fridge.

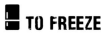 **TO FREEZE**

Place jars in the freezer for up to one year.

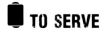 **TO SERVE**

Place jam in the refrigerator to thaw overnight.

AMOUNT PER SERVING: Calories 31.11; Total Fat 0.06 g; Cholesterol 0 mg; Sodium 1.78 mg; Potassium 17.03 mg; Total Carbohydrates 8.04 g; Fiber 0.68 g; Sugar 6.62 g; Protein 0.15 g

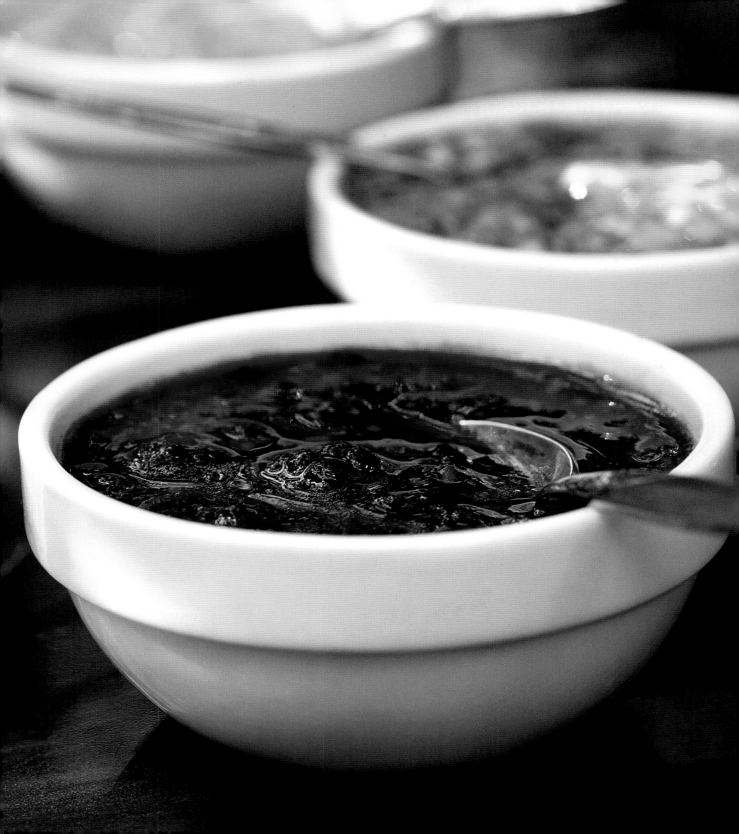

# ALL-PURPOSE ASIAN SPICE BLEND

This is a versatile spice blend that can be rubbed into meat and poultry, tossed with Asian noodles, whisked into sauces, used to crust fish, and blended with sesame oil and tamari for a dipping sauce.

½ cup (16 g) dried mint leaves

¼ cup (24 g) dried orange peel

3 tablespoons (24 g) white sesame seeds

2 tablespoons (6 g) dried lemongrass

1 teaspoon ground white pepper

¼ teaspoon salt

Pinch of cayenne

① Place all ingredients in a food processor and pulse to crush sesame seeds.

YIELD: 1 CUP (10 G)
SERVINGS: 48 (0.1 OUNCE)

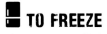 **TO FREEZE**

Place in a 1-quart (950 ml) freezer bag or freezer-safe container.

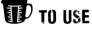 **TO USE**

Portion out the amount needed.

AMOUNT PER SERVING: Calories 3.81; Total Fat 0.25 g; Cholesterol 0 mg; Sodium 12.28 mg; Potassium 5.88 mg; Total Carbohydrates 0.35 g; Fiber 0.15 g; Sugar 0 g; Protein 0.11 g

# WHOLE-GRAIN BREAD CRUMBS

Dried bread crumbs are a kitchen staple for many yummy dishes, including meatloaf, breading for chicken and fish, or toasted with a little butter or olive oil and sprinkled on pasta or vegetables. Sure, you can pick up a package of store-bought bread crumbs, but making your own is a snap and gives you the opportunity to use up day-old bread, saving you money and reducing food waste.

**1 loaf Zesty Garlic Rosemary Bread (page 126) or 1 (16-ounce, or 455 g) loaf whole-grain bread**

① Preheat oven to 200°F (93°C, or gas mark under ½).

② Tear or cut bread into same-size chunks and spread on a large rimmed baking sheet.

③ Bake for 20 minutes or until they are thoroughly dried out and turning a bit golden. Remove from the oven and allow to cool completely.

④ Place bread in a food processor and pulse a few times to break down chunks. Turn processor on high and process just until you get a crumb consistency.

YIELD: 4 CUPS (460 G)
SERVINGS: 64 (0.3 OUNCE)

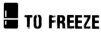 **TO FREEZE**

Place crumbs in 1-quart (950 ml) freezer bags.

 **TO USE**

Remove the amount of bread crumbs you need.

AMOUNT PER SERVING: Calories 18.84; Total Fat 0.3 g; Cholesterol 0 mg; Sodium 29.86mg; Potassium 16.35 mg; Total Carbohydrates 3.08 g; Fiber0.53 g; Sugar 0.45 g; Protein 0.95 g

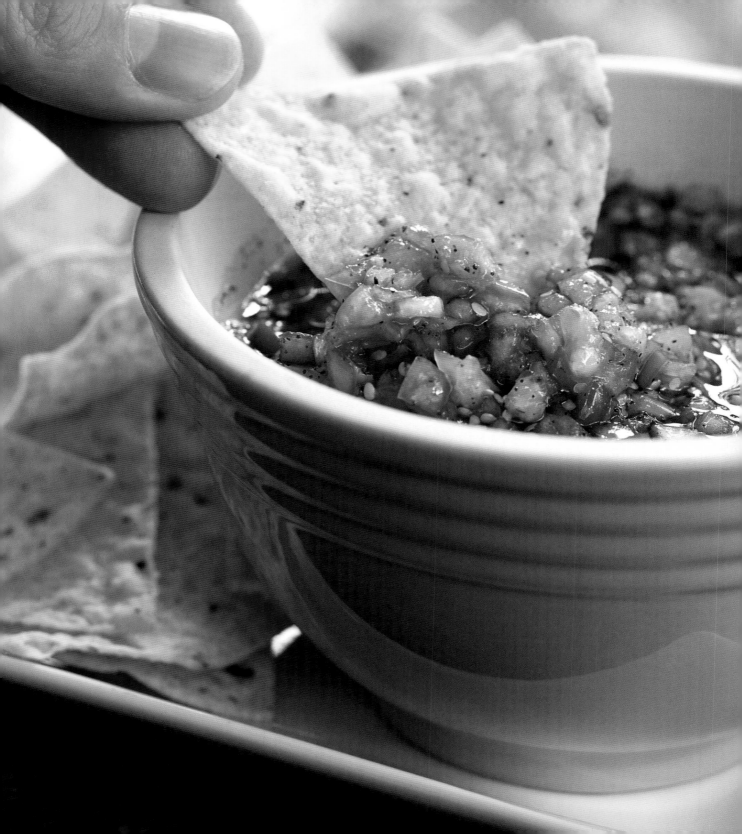

# SAVORY TOMATILLO JAM

Tomatillos, those often overlooked fruits used like a vegetable, resemble a green tomato wrapped in a husk. Popular in Mexican cuisine, tomatillos effortlessly become a thick sauce in this sweet and savory jam recipe. Naturally low in calories, tomatillos are a good source of vitamin C. Try the jam with Black Bean Breakfast Burritos (page 184) or Lean, Mean Mexican Turkey and Rice Casserole (page 25).

**2 packages (1.59 ounces, or 45 g) freezer jam fruit pectin**

**3 cups (600 g) granulated sugar**

**8 cups (1.1 kg) husked, finely chopped tomatillos**

**Grated zest of 1 lime**

**Juice of 2 limes**

**2 jalapeños, halved, seeded (or not), finely chopped**

**1½ teaspoons chipotle powder**

**10 plastic freezer jars (8 ounces, or 235 g, each)**

(1) In a large bowl, stir together pectin and sugar.

(2) Add tomatillos, lime zest, lime juice, jalapeños, and chipotle powder. Stir well to combine.

(3) Using a funnel, spoon jam into freezer jars to fill line. Twist on lids. Let stand for 30 minutes or until thickened.

YIELD: TEN 8-OUNCE (227 G) JARS
SERVINGS SIZE: 1 TABLESPOON, OR 20 G

## SERVING SUGGESTIONS

Tomatillo jam is a savory-sweet condiment that will delectably spice up your everyday meals. Try it spread on corn bread for breakfast, pour it over a block of cream cheese or goat cheese to make a dip for baked chips, use it in place of salsa for your Mexican meals, or simply substitute it for mayonnaise or mustard when making wraps and sandwiches.

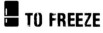 **TO FREEZE**

Place jars in the freezer for up to one year.

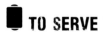 **TO SERVE**

Place jam in the refrigerator to thaw overnight.

AMOUNT PER SERVING: Calories 25.13; Total Fat 0.09 g; Cholesterol 0 mg; Sodium 1.69 mg; Potassium 8.9 mg; Total Carbohydrates 6.5 g; Fiber 0.16 g; Sugar 5.58 g; Protein 0.04 g

# CHAPTER 10

# BREAKFASTS
## HEALTHY CHOICES AS YOU'RE HEADING OUT THE DOOR

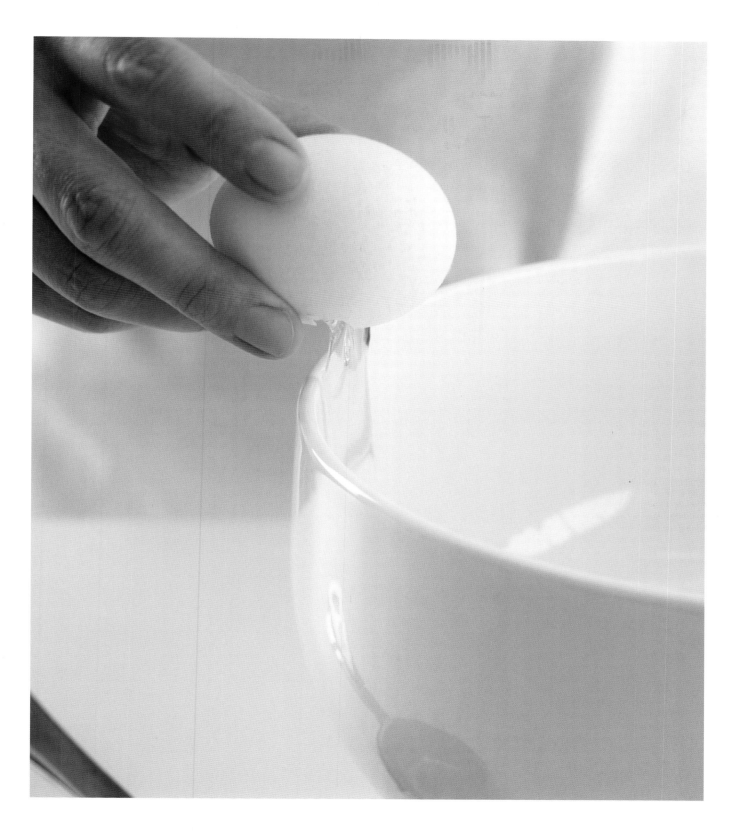

# QUICK AND EASY ENGLISH MUFFIN TOASTER WAFFLES

If your waffle iron has been gathering dust because you don't want to deal with waffle batter mess, you'll love this waffle-making shortcut. No need to worry about botched waffles sticking to the iron—this English muffin version delivers perfect "waffles" every time. Best yet, they freeze easily and can be popped into the toaster for a healthy breakfast far superior than frozen waffles out of a box. They're also especially yummy topped with Spicy Blackberry Freezer Jam (page 172).

**6 eggs**

**1¼ cups (285 ml) milk**

**1 teaspoon ground cinnamon**

**1 teaspoon grated orange zest**

**1 teaspoon pure vanilla extract**

**8 whole-grain English muffins, split in half**

1. Preheat waffle iron.

2. In a large, wide, shallow dish, whisk together eggs, milk, cinnamon, orange zest, and vanilla.

3. Spray waffle iron with nonstick cooking spray or brush with oil. Dip English muffin halves in egg mixture and arrange 2 to 4 (or however many will fit) on the waffle iron. Close lid, pressing down slightly, and cook until English muffins are golden brown and egg mixture has set.

4. Transfer to a wire rack to cool completely. Repeat with remaining egg batter and English muffins.

YIELD: 16 WAFFLES, OR 8 SERVINGS

## NUTRITION TIP: WHY BREAKFAST RULES

Your mom was right—breakfast *is* the most important meal of the day. Skipping breakfast not only saps your energy, it puts you at risk of making poor food choices and overeating later in the day. If you're a parent, you should know this: Hungry kids have trouble concentrating and don't perform academically or on the playground as well as kids who start the day with a morning meal.

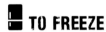 ## TO FREEZE

Place in a single layer on a baking sheet and freeze until solid. Transfer to a 1-gallon (3.8 L) freezer bag, removing as much air as possible before sealing.

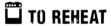 ## TO REHEAT

MICROWAVE METHOD: Remove frozen waffle from freezer and place on a microwave-safe plate. Microwave at 50% power for 2 minutes or until heated through.

TOASTER METHOD: Place frozen waffle in toaster and toast until heated through and crisp.

AMOUNT PER SERVING: Calories 229.49; Total Fat 5.67 g; Cholesterol 161.67 mg; Sodium 342.71 mg; Potassium 211.56 mg; Total Carbohydrates 32.76 g; Fiber 1.87 g; Sugar 2.81 g; Protein 11.98 g

# OAT-RAGEOUS CINNAMON BROWN SUGAR WAFFLES

If you're a waffle purist, carve out a morning to make a double or triple batch of these sweet and hearty whole-grain treats. Waffles freeze well and can be on the table in minutes after a reheat in the toaster or oven, tasting just as fresh as they did straight off the iron. Serve with Spicy Blackberry Freezer Jam (page 172).

¾ cup (60 g) rolled oats

1¼ cups (156 g) whole-wheat flour

1 cup (125 g) all-purpose flour

3 tablespoons (41 g) nonfat dry milk powder

1 teaspoon ground cinnamon

½ teaspoon ground allspice

¼ cup (60 g) packed brown sugar

1 teaspoon salt

1½ tablespoons (21 g) baking powder

1½ tablespoons (21 g) baking soda

2 eggs

2¼ cups (535 ml) nonfat buttermilk

3 tablespoons (42 g) unsalted butter, melted

① Preheat waffle iron. Place oats in a food processor and process for 30 seconds or until coarsely ground. Add flours, milk powder, cinnamon, allspice, brown sugar, salt, baking powder, and baking soda. Pulse until well-combined.

② In a large bowl, whisk together eggs, buttermilk, and butter until smooth. Add flour mixture and whisk until well-combined.

③ Generously spray waffle iron with cooking spray. Pour about 1½ cups (355 ml) batter (or however much your iron holds) onto the center of the waffle iron. Close lid and cook until waffles are golden and cooked through. Transfer to a wire rack to cool completely. Repeat with remaining batter.

YIELD: 12 WAFFLES, OR 6 SERVINGS

## COOKING TIP: TRY WHITE WHOLE-WHEAT FLOUR

If you find the heartiness of whole-wheat flour undesirable, give white whole-wheat flour a try. Lighter in texture and milder in flavor, white whole-wheat flour bakes similarly to all-purpose flour yet provides the same nutrition as whole-wheat flour. Most of the recipes in this book call for both all-purpose and whole-wheat flour. However, you can use 100% white whole-wheat flour if desired. There is one exception: Do not substitute white whole-wheat flour for whole-wheat pastry flour, since white whole-wheat flour has a higher protein percentage.

 **TO FREEZE**

Place waffles on a baking sheet in one layer and freeze until firm. Transfer to a 1-gallon (3.8 L) freezer bag, removing as much air as possible before sealing.

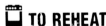 **TO REHEAT**

TOASTER METHOD: Place frozen waffles in toaster and toast until heated through and crisp.

OVEN METHOD: Preheat oven to 350°F (180°C, or gas mark 4). Place waffles on a baking sheet and bake for 10 minutes or until heated through.

AMOUNT PER SERVING: Calories 393.41; Total Fat 10.56 g; Cholesterol 94.17 mg; Sodium 1862.51 mg; Potassium 451.93 mg; Total Carbohydrates 123.24 g; Fiber 4.99 g; Sugar 18.59 g; Protein 15.45 g

# SALMON CREAM CHEESE BREAKFAST BURRITOS

Salmon, cream cheese, and garlic-kissed spinach wrapped in a whole-grain tortilla is a breakfast abundant in omega-3s, antioxidants, vitamins A and K, magnesium, folic acid, and fiber. These burritos are a tasty way to sneak more leafy greens into your family's diet.

**1 tablespoon (15 ml) olive oil**

**1 clove garlic, minced**

**8 cups (240 g) baby spinach**

**1 bunch scallions, chopped (white and green parts)**

**2 packages (8 ounces, or 225 g, each) cream cheese, softened at room temperature**

**1¾ pounds (795 g) cooked salmon, flaked, cooled**

**10 (8-inch, or 20 cm) whole-grain flour tortillas**

① Heat oil in a Dutch oven over medium heat. Add garlic and cook, stirring, for 1 minute. Add spinach and scallions. Cook, stirring occasionally, for 4 minutes or until greens are wilted. Spread spinach mixture on paper towels to drain and cool.

② In a food processor, process cream cheese for 30 seconds or until smooth. Add spinach mixture and pulse to combine. Add salmon and pulse to combine.

③ Spread tortillas with salmon mixture, fold edges over, and roll burrito-style.

YIELD: 10 BURRITOS, OR 10 SERVINGS

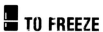 **TO FREEZE**

Wrap each burrito in freezer wrap or plastic wrap and place in 1-gallon (3.8 L) freezer bags, removing as much air as possible before sealing.

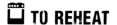 **TO REHEAT**

Thaw burritos in refrigerator overnight.

MICROWAVE METHOD: Unwrap burritos and place on a microwave-safe plate. Reheat on high for 1 minute or until heated through. If you forget to thaw burritos, microwave frozen burritos at 50% power for 2 to 3 minutes or until heated through.

OVEN METHOD: Preheat oven to 375°F (190°C, or gas mark 5). Unwrap burritos and place them side by side in a baking dish. Cover with foil and reheat for 15 minutes or until heated through.

AMOUNT PER SERVING: Calories 423.35; Total Fat 29.12 g; Cholesterol 99.98 mg; Sodium 443.4 mg; Potassium 522 mg; Total Carbohydrates 14.91 g; Fiber 8.79 g; Sugar 2.43 g; Protein 24.88 g

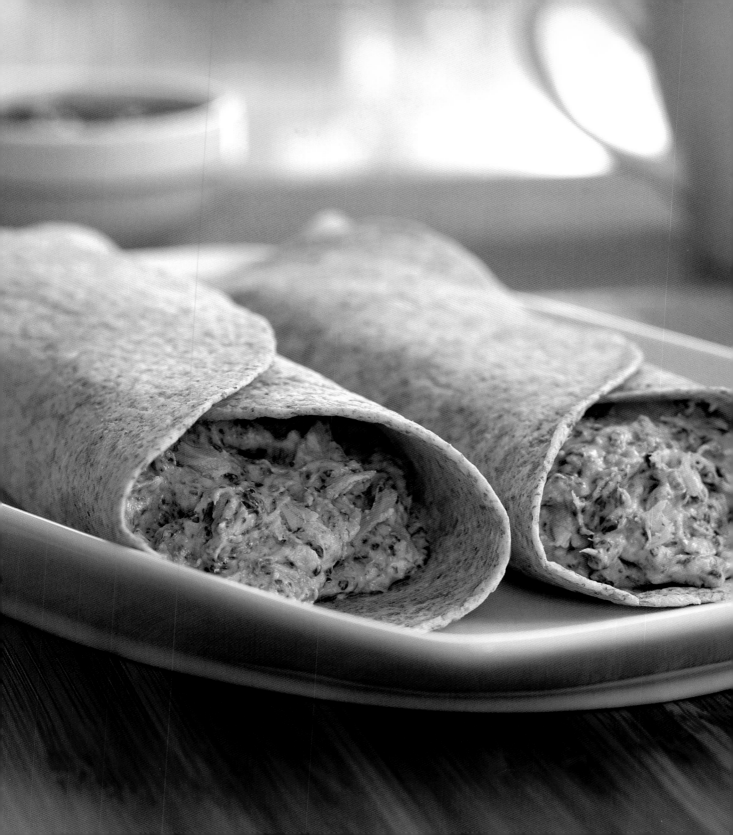

# BLACK BEAN BREAKFAST BURRITOS

Breakfast burritos can't be beat when it comes to a healthy, balanced morning meal. Having them ready to grab from the freezer or fridge not only gives you a tasty to-go meal, it's also a budget-friendly breakfast compared to drive-thru fare.

1 tablespoon (15 ml) canola oil

1 cup (160 g) finely chopped onion

1 cup (150 g) finely chopped red bell pepper

3 cloves garlic, minced

8 eggs, lightly beaten

1 can (15 ounces, or 425 g) black beans, rinsed, drained

⅓ cup (5 g) finely chopped fresh cilantro

10 (8-inch, or 20 cm) whole-grain flour tortillas

1¼ cups (144 g) shredded pepper jack cheese

① Heat oil in a large skillet over medium-high heat. Add onion and bell pepper and cook, stirring often, until vegetables are softened. Add garlic and cook, stirring, for 1 minute.

② Reduce heat to medium-low and add eggs, shaking the pan to distribute eggs. Let cook for 2 minutes and then use a spatula to flip and break up mixture. Continue to cook and occasionally stir until eggs are no longer liquidy.

③ Stir in black beans and cook just until heated through. Stir in cilantro and remove from heat and let cool.

④ Fill tortillas with black bean mixture and sprinkle with cheese. Fold edges of tortilla over filling and roll burrito-style.

YIELD: 10 BURRITOS, OR SERVINGS

 **TO FREEZE**

Wrap each burrito in freezer wrap or plastic wrap and place in 1-gallon (3.8 L) freezer bags, removing as much air as possible before sealing.

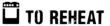 **TO REHEAT**

Thaw burritos in refrigerator overnight.

MICROWAVE METHOD: Unwrap burritos and place on a microwave-safe plate. Reheat on high for 1 minute or until heated through. If you forget to thaw burritos, microwave frozen burritos on 50% power for 2 to 3 minutes or until heated through.

OVEN METHOD: Preheat oven to 375°F (190°C, or gas mark 5). Unwrap burritos and place them side by side in a baking dish. Cover with foil and reheat for 15 minutes or until heated through.

AMOUNT PER SERVING: Calories 258.21; Total Fat 11.96 g; Cholesterol 182.02 mg; Sodium 451.28 mg; Potassium 240.92 mg; Total Carbohydrates 22.77 g; Fiber 11.43 g; Sugar 3.7 g; Protein 14.81 g

# QUICK-TO-THE-TABLE CHEESY SPINACH QUICHE

Quiche is always an impressive breakfast or brunch dish for guests but is no more difficult to make than an omelet. Instead of reserving quiche for special occasions, keep a variety in the freezer and you'll have a yummy 30-minute morning meal that you can serve any day of the week. This recipe features spinach, but you can easily swap it out for arugula, chard, kale, and beet or mustard greens (heartier leafies will take a little longer to cook).

**Double-Crust Whole-Wheat Pie Dough (page 204), omit sugar**

**1 tablespoon (15 ml) olive oil**

**¼ cup (40 g) finely chopped shallots**

**4 cups (120 g) baby spinach leaves, chopped**

**Kosher salt and freshly ground black pepper to taste**

**8 eggs**

**1½ cups (355 ml) milk**

**1½ cups (355 ml) half-and-half**

**1 teaspoon dried thyme**

**Pinch of cayenne**

**¼ teaspoon freshly grated nutmeg**

**8 ounces (225 g) grated Gruyère cheese**

① Preheat oven to 350°F (180°C, or gas mark 4). Roll 2 portions of pie dough out and line two (9-inch, or 23 cm) pie plates. Place in the refrigerator.

② In a large skillet over medium heat, heat oil and cook shallot, stirring often, until softened and translucent. Add spinach and cook, stirring often, until wilted. Season with salt and pepper. Drain in a colander, pressing to remove liquid.

③ In a large bowl, whisk together eggs, milk, half-and-half, thyme, cayenne, and nutmeg. Divide spinach evenly between the 2 pie plates. Cover spinach with egg mixture. Sprinkle each with cheese. Gently shake pie plates to distribute egg mixture and cheese.

④ Place pie plates on a baking sheet in the oven. Bake for 55 minutes or until quiche is just set. Remove from the oven and let cool completely on wire racks.

YIELD: TWO 9-INCH (23 CM) QUICHES, OR 12 SERVINGS

## NUTRITION SPOTLIGHT: LEAFY GREENS

Vitamin-packed leafy greens are loaded with nutrition. Here are some more ways to incorporate them into your diet:

- Add spinach, arugula, dandelion greens, or escarole to omelets or breakfast burritos.
- Include steamed or sautéed chard or kale in lasagna or enchiladas.
- Sauté any leafy green with olive oil and garlic for a super-nutritious side dish.
- Purée tender greens with light mayonnaise or Neufchâtel for a dip.
- Toss spinach and other salad greens into a bowl with toasted nuts, currants, and a balsamic vinaigrette.

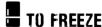 **TO FREEZE**

INDIVIDUAL SERVINGS: Cut each quiche into 6 portions and transfer to individual serving-size freezer- and microwave-safe containers.

FOR A CROWD: Place quiche in the freezer on a baking sheet until firm. Tightly wrap with freezer wrap or plastic wrap and heavy-duty aluminum foil. Stack and slide into a 1-gallon (3.8 L) freezer bag.

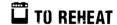 **TO REHEAT**

For individual servings, let quiche thaw in refrigerator overnight. If serving a crowd, do not thaw whole quiche before reheating.

MICROWAVE METHOD: Reheat individual servings of quiche in the microwave on 60% power for 2 minutes or until heated through.

OVEN METHOD: Preheat oven to 350°F (180°C, or gas mark 4). Place whole quiche uncovered on a baking sheet and reheat in the oven for 30 minutes or until heated through.

AMOUNT PER SERVING: Calories 195.74; Total Fat 14.72 g; Cholesterol 175.45 mg; Sodium 143.54 mg; Potassium 213.15 mg; Total Carbohydrates 4.07 g; Fiber 0.27 g; Sugar 1.97 g; Protein 12.12 g

# OMEGA-3 SMOKED SALMON OMELET

A protein-rich breakfast boasting omega-3s, this omelet is loaded with flavor. In addition to the healthy fats from the salmon, omega-3 eggs also provide a tasty dose of the heart-healthy fatty acids. Opt for eggs from local organic pasture-raised chickens, if possible, since research shows these eggs have double the omega-3s and vitamin E as compared to eggs from cage-raised chickens.

.........................................................................................................................................

**12 omega-3 eggs**

**2 cloves garlic, pressed**

**3 tablespoons (12 g) chopped fresh dill**

**3 tablespoons (9 g) chopped fresh chives**

**12 ounces (340 g) smoked sockeye salmon, flaked**

**1 cup (120 g) shredded Gruyère cheese**

**2 tablespoons (28 ml) olive oil**

**¾ cup (60 g) shredded Parmesan cheese**

① Preheat broiler. In a large bowl, lightly beat the eggs. Whisk in garlic, dill, chives, salmon, and Gruyère cheese.

② Heat oil in 2 large ovenproof skillets over medium-high heat. Divide egg mixture between the skillets and cook for 2 minutes. Reduce heat to low and cook 8 minutes or until eggs are almost set.

③ Sprinkle each omelet with Parmesan and set skillets under broiler for 1 to 2 minutes or until omelets are lightly browned. Cool completely.

YIELD: 2 LARGE OMELETS, OR 12 SERVINGS

## NUTRITION SPOTLIGHT: SALMON

Being a fatty fish, salmon is highly prized for its omega-3 fats, which are associated with a reduced risk of heart disease and inflammation, but it is also loaded with vitamin D, B vitamins, selenium, and magnesium. Eating salmon, preferably wild salmon, at least twice per week can decrease your risk of stroke, blood clots, diabetes, some types of cancers, arthritis, and Alzheimer's as well as boost your bone health and even improve your mental health.

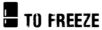 **TO FREEZE**

INDIVIDUAL SERVINGS: Cut each omelet into wedges. Place on a baking sheet and freeze until just solid. Wrap each wedge with freezer wrap or place in a freezer- and microwave-safe container.

FOR A CROWD: Place entire omelets on a baking sheet and freeze until just solid. Wrap tightly with freezer wrap.

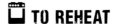 **TO REHEAT**

Let omelet wedges or entire omelets thaw in the refrigerator for a few hours.

MICROWAVE METHOD: Individual wedges can be microwaved on high for 2 minutes or until heated through.

STOVETOP METHOD: Set entire omelet in original skillet over medium heat. Set a lid on skillet and cook for 6 minutes or until heated through.

AMOUNT PER SERVING: Calories 120.08; Total Fat 5.42 g; Cholesterol 43.92 mg; Sodium 16.68 mg; Potassium 309.33 mg; Total Carbohydrates 0.76 g; Fiber 0.17 g; Sugar 0.02 g; Protein 17.43 g

# BROCCOLI AND GOAT CHEESE ON-THE-GO OMELET

Broccoli and goat cheese are a delicious pair in this satisfying breakfast dish. There's no broccoli on hand? Substitute cauliflower or sliced brussels sprouts. You're not a fan of goat cheese? Swap it out for feta. Omelets lend themselves to many mouthwatering variations.

**3 tablespoons (45 ml) olive oil**

**6 cups (426 g) chopped broccoli florets**

**Salt and freshly ground black pepper to taste**

**2 cloves garlic, minced**

**12 eggs**

**3 tablespoons (12 g) finely chopped parsley**

**1 cup (150 g) crumbled goat cheese**

① Heat oil in a 12-inch (30 cm) skillet over medium heat. Add broccoli and cook, stirring often, until broccoli is tender and lightly browned. Season with salt and pepper and add garlic and cook, stirring, for 1 minute more.

② In a large bowl, beat eggs. Whisk in parsley and goat cheese. Pour egg mixture over broccoli and shake skillet to let egg mixture run under broccoli. Cook, shaking skillet occasionally, until eggs are just set.

③ Slide omelet onto a large plate. Set skillet upside down over plate. Using oven mitts, grab skillet and plate and invert omelet back into skillet and cook 1 minute more. Slide onto a plate and cool completely.

YIELD: 8 SERVINGS

## NUTRITION SPOTLIGHT: THE BRASSICA FAMILY

Broccoli, along with broccoli rabe, cauliflower, brussels sprouts, cabbage, bok choy, turnips, and kale, is part of the Brassica family, also known as cruciferous vegetables. Though the crucifers are considered superfoods, they may have a negative effect on thyroid function in large quantities, so be sure to include a wide variety of vegetables in your diet.

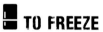 **TO FREEZE**

INDIVIDUAL SERVINGS: Cut omelet into 8 wedges and place on a baking sheet. Freeze until just solid and then wrap each with freezer wrap.

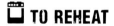 **TO REHEAT**

Let omelet wedges or entire omelet thaw in the refrigerator for a few hours.

MICROWAVE METHOD: Individual wedges can be microwaved on high for 2 minutes or until heated through.

STOVETOP METHOD: Place entire omelet in original skillet over medium heat. Cover with a lid and cook for 5 to 6 minutes or until heated through.

AMOUNT PER SERVING: Calories 219.11; Total Fat 16.74 g; Cholesterol 325.88 mg; Sodium 188.89 mg; Potassium 284.27 mg; Total Carbohydrates 3.81 g; Fiber 0.03 g; Sugar 0.76 g; Protein 14.56 g

# WHOLE-GRAIN RAISIN BREAD AND SAUSAGE BAKE

Far healthier than the drive-thru egg-and-sausage sandwiches, this breakfast casserole is loaded with flavor yet light on fat, sodium, and calories.

2 tablespoons (28 ml) canola oil

1 pound (455 g) low-fat chicken sausage, casings removed, crumbled

8 eggs

4 cups (950 ml) 2% milk

Pinch of salt

A few grinds black pepper

1 loaf (1 pound, or 455 g) whole-grain raisin bread, cut into strips

Maple syrup

① Heat oil in a skillet over medium heat and cook sausage, stirring occasionally, until browned. Set aside to cool. In a large bowl, whisk together eggs and milk. Add salt and pepper.

② Grease a 13 x 9-inch (33 x 23 cm) baking dish. Arrange half of the bread in the bottom of prepared dish. Sprinkle half of the sausage over bread. Layer remaining bread over sausage. Sprinkle with remaining sausage.

③ Pour egg mixture over bread and shake dish to distribute egg throughout. Press bread down and set aside to soak for 30 minutes or cover and place in refrigerator overnight.

④ Preheat oven to 350°F (180°C, or gas mark 4). Set baking dish on a baking sheet and bake for 1 hour or until set. Let cool completely on a wire rack (if you are freezing these as individual servings, cut into serving sizes to cool quicker).

YIELD: 8 SERVINGS

## NUTRITION TIP: FIBER UP

For a flavorful fiber boost, substitute sprouted whole-grain bread or whole-wheat bread for white bread in your everyday recipes. To up your family's fiber intake, serve whole fruits and vegetables instead of fruit and vegetable juices, buy whole-grain products with at least 3 grams of fiber per serving, and limit refined white flour products in your family's meals and snacks.

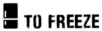 ## TO FREEZE

INDIVIDUAL SERVINGS: Cut casserole into 8 squares. Set on a baking sheet and allow to freeze until just solid. Wrap each in freezer wrap.

FOR A CROWD: Wrap baking dish with freezer wrap.

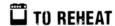 ## TO REHEAT

Let casserole thaw in refrigerator overnight.

MICROWAVE METHOD: Individual servings can be reheated in microwave on high for 2 minutes or until heated through.

OVEN METHOD: Preheat oven to 350°F (180°C, or gas mark 4). Remove freezer wrap and bake for 25 minutes or until heated through.

AMOUNT PER SERVING: Calories 255.59; Total Fat 12.2 g; Cholesterol 231.84 mg; Sodium 285.13 mg; Potassium 250.71 mg; Total Carbohydrates 21.37 g; Fiber 0.69 g; Sugar 11.76 g; Protein 14.8 g

# GINGERY SOUR CREAM COFFEE CAKE

The intoxicating aroma of a gingery cinnamon coffee cake baking in your oven is enough to bring the pickiest breakfast eaters to the table. As a bonus, home-baked coffee cake is a big winner over the store-bought coffee cakes laden with high fructose corn syrup and trans fats. Moist, delicious, and perfect for everyday and special occasions, keeping a few of these coffee cakes in the freezer means you'll always have an easy go-to morning nibble.

FOR THE CAKE:

½ cup (112 g) unsalted butter, softened at room temperature

⅔ cup (133 g) granulated sugar

2 eggs

2 teaspoons pure vanilla extract

¾ cup (72 g) finely chopped crystallized ginger

1 cup (120 g) whole-wheat pastry flour

1 cup (125 g) all-purpose flour

1 teaspoon baking soda

1 teaspoon baking powder

½ teaspoon salt

1 cup (230 g) light sour cream

FOR THE TOPPING:

3 tablespoons (23 g) whole-wheat pastry flour

⅔ cup (150 g) firmly packed brown sugar

1 tablespoon (7 g) ground cinnamon

½ teaspoon ground ginger

½ teaspoon freshly ground nutmeg

Pinch of ground cloves

3 tablespoons (42 g) butter, melted

¾ cup (83 g) coarsely chopped pecans

① Preheat oven to 350°F (180°C, or gas mark 4). Grease an 8-inch (20 cm) square baking pan. Cover the bottom of the pan with a piece of parchment or waxed paper.

② In the bowl of a standup mixer fitted with the paddle attachment, cream butter and sugar until fluffy. Add eggs, one at a time, beating well after each addition. Mix in vanilla and crystallized ginger.

③ In a medium bowl, whisk together flours, baking soda, baking powder, and salt. Add flour mixture to butter mixture, alternating with sour cream. Mix until well-combined. Pour batter into prepared baking pan.

④ In a small bowl, combine topping ingredients. Sprinkle topping evenly over batter.

⑤ Bake for 30 to 35 minutes or until a cake tester inserted in the center comes out clean. Cool cake in pan on a wire rack for 15 minutes. Loosen sides of cake with a knife. Invert cake onto a large plate and then back to the wire rack to cool completely crumb-side up.

YIELD: 16 SERVINGS

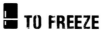 **TO FREEZE**

Tightly wrap cake in freezer wrap or plastic wrap and a sheet of heavy-duty aluminum foil.

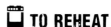 **TO REHEAT**

Remove foil and allow cake to thaw at room temperature. Preheat oven to 325°F (170°C, or gas mark 3). Remove foil and plastic from cake and place on a baking sheet. Bake for 10 to 15 minutes or until warmed through.

AMOUNT PER SERVING: Calories 307.95; Total Fat 14.08 g; Cholesterol 52.74 mg; Sodium 207.49 mg; Potassium 84.73 mg; Total Carbohydrates 42.71 g; Fiber 1.48 g; Sugar 26.93 g; Protein 3.57g

# PROSCIUTTO, ARTICHOKE, AND TOMATO STRATA

A mouthwatering Mediterranean meal, layers of flavorful prosciutto, tangy feta, tender artichoke hearts, and meaty sun-dried tomatoes make this strata a memorable way to start the day.

3 cups (700 ml) 2% milk, divided

¼ cup (60 ml) olive oil

8 cups (400 g) 1-inch (2.5 cm) cubes cracked wheat sourdough bread, crusts trimmed

½ cup (120 ml) half-and-half

6 eggs

1 tablespoon (10 g) chopped garlic

1 teaspoon salt

Freshly ground black pepper to taste

8 ounces (225 g) feta cheese, crumbled

2 tablespoons (6 g) chopped fresh sage

1 tablespoon (4 g) chopped fresh thyme

6 ounces (170 g) thinly sliced prosciutto

2 jars (6.5 ounces, or 185 g) marinated artichoke hearts, drained, coarsely chopped

2 cups (220 g) sun-dried tomatoes packed in olive oil, coarsely chopped

1 cup (110 g) shredded fontina cheese

1 cup (80 g) shredded Parmesan cheese

① Preheat oven to 350°F (180°C, or gas mark 4) and grease a 13 x 9-inch (33 x 23 cm) baking dish.

② In a large bowl, whisk together 2 cups (475 ml) milk and oil in large bowl. Add bread cubes and let soak for 10 minutes.

③ In a large bowl, whisk remaining milk and half-and-half together. Whisk in eggs, garlic, salt, and pepper. Stir in feta and herbs.

④ Place half of the bread mixture in prepared baking dish. Layer with half of the prosciutto. Top with half of the artichoke hearts, sun-dried tomatoes, and cheeses. Pour half of the egg mixture over, shaking dish to distribute it.

⑤ Repeat layering with bread mixture, prosciutto, artichoke hearts, tomatoes, and cheeses. Cover with remaining egg mixture, shaking dish to distribute. Set aside to soak for 30 minutes.

⑥ Bake strata uncovered for 1 hour or until set. Cool on a wire rack (if you are freezing as individual servings, cut into serving sizes to cool quicker).

YIELD: 12 SERVINGS

## NUTRITION SPOTLIGHT: EGGS

In addition to being nature's perfect muscle-building protein, one large egg contains 13 essential vitamins and minerals, healthy unsaturated fats, antioxidants, and a mere 70 calories! Eggs are rich in choline, an amino acid that boosts brain function, are associated with healthy fetal development, and help break down homocysteine, which is linked to heart disease. Eggs also promote eye health and ward off macular degeneration because they contain lutein and zeaxanthin, two antioxidants found in egg yolks.

AMOUNT PER SERVING: Calories 404.69; Total Fat 22.36 g; Cholesterol 157.55 mg; Sodium 1246.80 mg; Potassium 638.47 mg; Total Carbohydrates 30.84 g; Fiber 4.10 g; Sugar 4.94 g; Protein 22.34 g

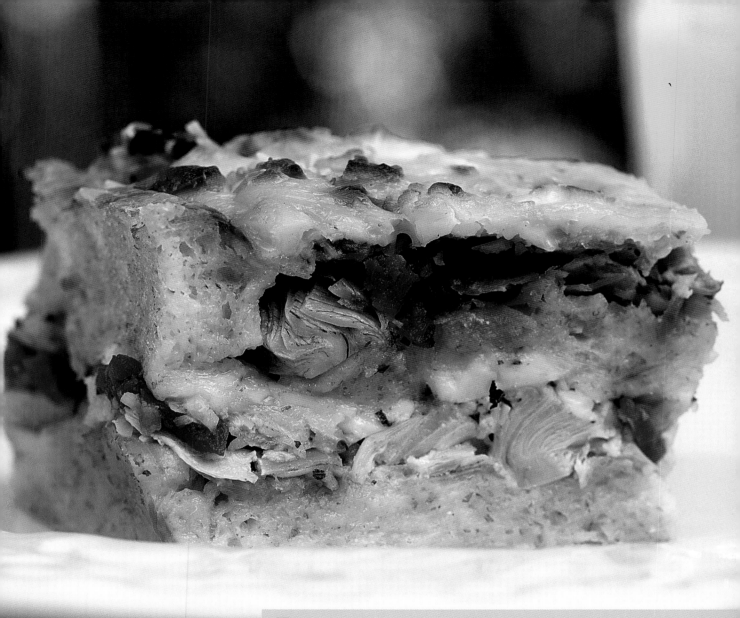

## TO FREEZE

INDIVIDUAL SERVINGS: Cut strata into 8 squares and place on a baking sheet. Freeze until just solid. Wrap each serving with freezer wrap.

FOR A CROWD: Wrap baking dish with freezer wrap.

## TO REHEAT

Let strata thaw in the refrigerator overnight.

MICROWAVE METHOD: Individual servings can be microwaved on high for 2 minutes or until heated through.

OVEN METHOD: Preheat oven to 350°F (180°C, or gas mark 4). Bake strata uncovered for 25 to 30 minutes or until heated through.

# RASPBERRY-LAVENDER CRUMB CAKE

Edible flowers are becoming popular additions to cocktails, salads, and desserts in many upscale restaurants, but you don't have to find a four-star eatery to enjoy their floral essence. Culinary lavender buds, along with many other edible flowers, are increasingly available at natural foods stores and can also be ordered online. They lend their lovely floral flavor and scent to this stunning berry crumb cake.

**FOR THE CAKE:**

**¼ cup (55 g) unsalted butter, at room temperature**

**⅓ cup (115 g) agave nectar**

**2 eggs**

**½ cup (120 ml) milk**

**2 cups (240 g) whole-wheat pastry flour**

**3 teaspoons (13.8 g) baking powder**

**¼ teaspoon salt**

**2 cups (250 g) fresh raspberries**

**1 cup (110 g) slivered almonds**

**2 tablespoons (5 g) lavender buds, minced**

**FOR THE CRUMB TOPPING:**

**1 cup (225 g) firmly packed brown sugar**

**2 tablespoons (16 g) whole-wheat pastry flour**

**½ cup (112 g) unsalted butter, chilled, cut into pieces**

**1 teaspoon ground cinnamon**

**1 teaspoon freshly grated nutmeg**

① Preheat oven to 375°F (190°C, or gas mark 5). Grease and flour a 9-inch (23 cm) cake pan.

② In a standup mixer fitted with the paddle attachment, beat butter and agave until light and fluffy. Add eggs, one at a time, beating well after each addition. Beat in the milk.

③ In a small bowl, whisk together flour, baking powder, and salt. Add to butter mixture and blend well. Gently fold in raspberries, almonds, and lavender. Pour batter into prepared pan.

④ In a food processor, combine topping ingredients. Pulse to combine. Sprinkle over batter. Bake for 40 minutes or until a cake tester inserted in the center comes out clean. Let cool completely and remove from the pan.

YIELD: ONE 9-INCH (23 CM) CAKE, OR 10 SERVINGS

## COOKING TIP: FREEZE FRESH RASPBERRIES

Stocking up on berries and freezing them is the best way to preserve their fresh flavor and antioxidant-rich powers. Here's how to freeze raspberries: Place berries in a colander and gently rinse them under cool water. Spread them out on a stack of paper towels, gingerly pat them dry, and allow to air-dry. Spread them onto a rimmed baking sheet in a single layer and place them in the freezer until solid. Transfer to a large freezer bag.

AMOUNT PER SERVING: Calories 434.18; Total Fat 20.72 g; Cholesterol 79.19 mg; Sodium 232.58 mg; Potassium 211.84 mg; Total Carbohydrates 57.86 g; Fiber 4.41 g; Sugar 32.43 g; Protein 7.24 g

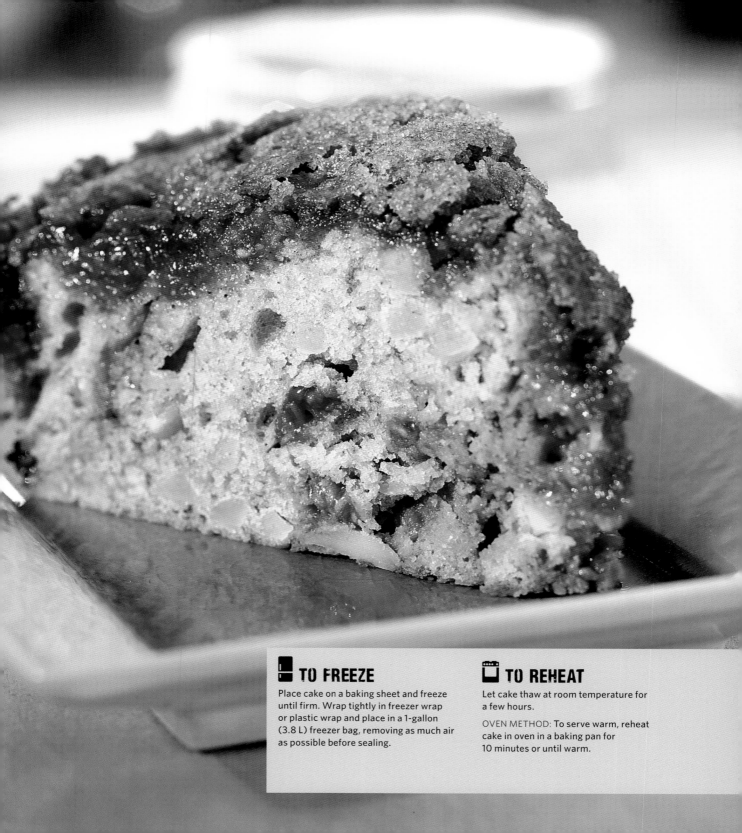

## TO FREEZE

Place cake on a baking sheet and freeze until firm. Wrap tightly in freezer wrap or plastic wrap and place in a 1-gallon (3.8 L) freezer bag, removing as much air as possible before sealing.

## TO REHEAT

Let cake thaw at room temperature for a few hours.

OVEN METHOD: To serve warm, reheat cake in oven in a baking pan for 10 minutes or until warm.

# BETTER-FOR-YOU BANANA SPICE BREAD

For an added health benefit, omega-3–rich flax is used in place of eggs. If you don't have ground flax on hand, simply substitute 2 large eggs.

**2 tablespoons ground (14 g) flax plus 6 tablespoons (90 ml) water**

**⅓ cup (67 g) granulated sugar**

**2 tablespoons (28 g) unsalted butter**

**1½ teaspoons pure vanilla extract**

**⅔ cup (154 g) plain yogurt**

**¾ cup (94 g) all-purpose flour**

**¾ cup (90 g) whole-wheat flour**

**½ teaspoon sea salt**

**1 teaspoon baking powder**

**1 teaspoon baking soda**

**1 teaspoon ground cinnamon**

**½ teaspoon ground allspice**

**½ teaspoon ground ginger**

**3 medium very ripe bananas, peeled, cut into chunks**

① Preheat oven to 375°F (190°C, or gas mark 5). Grease a 9-inch (23 cm) cake pan.

② Whisk together flax and water and set aside for 5 minutes. In a standup mixer, cream sugar and butter. Add flax mixture, vanilla, and yogurt and blend until smooth.

③ In a mixing bowl, whisk together flours, salt, baking powder, baking soda, and spices. Add flour mixture to yogurt mixture and blend on low until ingredients are just moist.

④ Add bananas and blend on low until incorporated, taking care not to mash bananas. Pour into cake pan and bake for about 25 minutes or until bread just turns golden and springs back when touched. Cool completely on a wire rack.

YIELD: ONE 9-INCH (23 CM) ROUND, OR 8 SERVINGS

## NUTRITION SPOTLIGHT: FLAX

Flax is not only loaded with vitamins, minerals, healthy fats, and fiber; it is a versatile ingredient. Research indicates that flax can reduce the risk of heart disease, cancer, stroke, diabetes, and some immune disorders due to its high level of omega-3 fatty acids, lignans, and fiber. However, to unleash the benefits of this tiny but powerful seed, you need to grind it or buy it in ground form. Aim for 1 tablespoon (7 g) of ground flax per day.

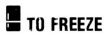 **TO FREEZE**

Tightly wrap bread in freezer wrap.

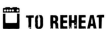 **TO REHEAT**

Let bread thaw at room temperature.

OVEN METHOD: To serve warm, place bread back in the 9-inch (23 cm) cake pan and reheat in a 350°F (180°C, or gas mark 4) oven.

AMOUNT PER SERVING:  Calories 204.86; Total Fat 4.37 g; Cholesterol 8.68 mg; Sodium 351.63 mg; Potassium 283.35 mg; Total Carbohydrates 38.47 g; Fiber 3.58 g; Sugar 15.36 g; Protein 4.69 g

# BAKED GINGERBREAD CAKE DOUGHNUTS WITH MAPLE GLAZE

Though a run to the doughnut shop or packaged breakfast foods aisle at the supermarket may seem a convenient move, those fried, heavily glazed goodies are laden with calories, unhealthy fats, and sugar. Baked doughnuts are not only a healthier choice for the family, they are fun to make with the kids and are quick to the table even after freezing.

## FOR THE DOUGHNUTS:

1½ cups (188 g) all-purpose flour

1½ cups (180 g) whole-wheat pastry flour

1 tablespoon (13.8 g) baking powder

½ teaspoon salt

⅔ cup (150 g) firmly packed brown sugar

½ teaspoon freshly ground nutmeg

1 teaspoon ground cinnamon

2 tablespoons (12 g) minced candied ginger

2 eggs

⅓ cup (75 g) unsalted butter, melted

1 tablespoon (20 g) molasses

½ cup (120 ml) milk

## FOR THE GLAZE:

1 cup (200 g) granulated sugar

¼ cup (80 g) maple syrup

1½ cups (355 ml) water

2 teaspoons pure vanilla extract

① In a large bowl, whisk together flours, baking powder, salt, brown sugar, nutmeg, cinnamon, and candied ginger. Set aside.

② In a medium bowl, beat eggs, butter, molasses, and milk until well-combined. Stir butter mixture into flour mixture just until moistened. Cover and refrigerate for 1 hour.

③ Preheat oven to 325°F (170°C, or gas mark 3). Roll dough out on a lightly floured surface until ½-inch (1.3 cm) thick. Using a 3-inch (7.5 cm) doughnut cutter (or a 3-inch [7.5 cm] biscuit cutter and 1-inch [2.5 cm] round pastry cutter), cut dough into 18 doughnuts and doughnut holes.

④ Place on greased baking sheets and bake for 10 to 12 minutes. Let cool on baking sheets for 5 minutes and then use a spatula to transfer to wire racks to cool completely.

YIELD: 18 DOUGHNUTS AND DOUGHNUT HOLES, OR 18 SERVINGS

*Recipe continued on next page*

## NUTRITION SPOTLIGHT: WHOLE-WHEAT PASTRY FLOUR

Whole-wheat pastry flour is similar to refined white pastry flour in that its fine texture produces light, feathery baked goods. However, whole-wheat pastry flour isn't stripped of all of the bran and germ in whole wheat, so it gives baked goods a nutritional edge, providing more fiber and nutrients. If you are used to traditional all-purpose flour based recipes, try substituting half of the all-purpose with whole-wheat pastry flour.

AMOUNT PER SERVING: Calories 209.8; Total Fat 4.4 g; Cholesterol 33.01 mg; Sodium 160.81 mg; Potassium 110.25 mg; Total Carbohydrates 40.25 g; Fiber 1.65 g; Sugar 22.79 g; Protein 3.49 g

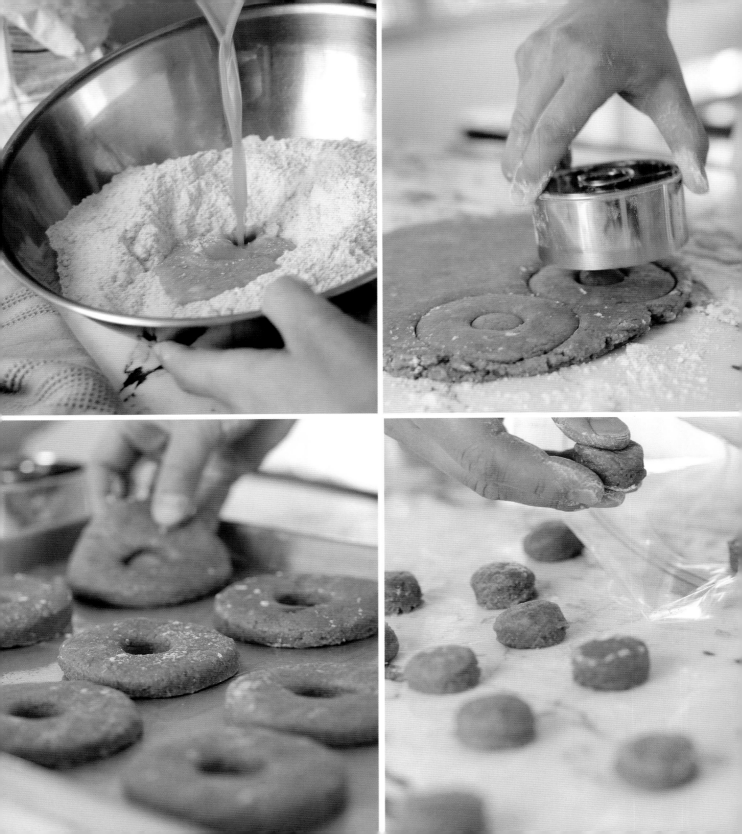

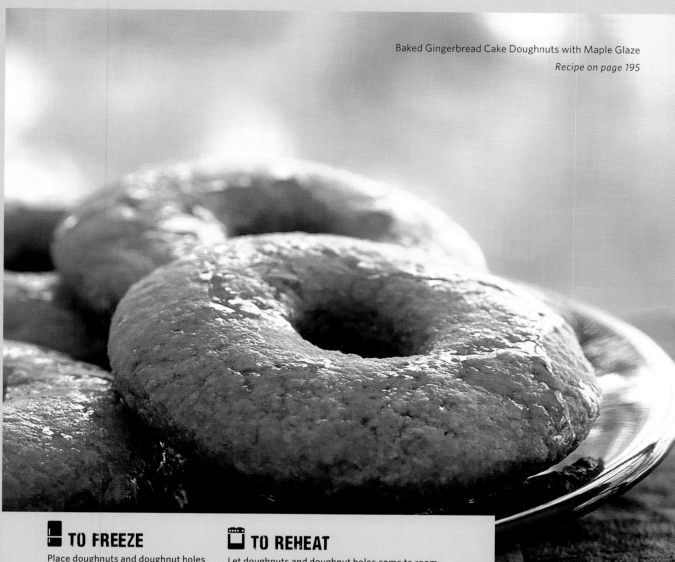

Baked Gingerbread Cake Doughnuts with Maple Glaze

*Recipe on page 195*

## 🧊 TO FREEZE

Place doughnuts and doughnut holes on baking sheets and freeze until solid. Place in a 1-gallon (3.8 L) freezer bag.

As an option, you can make doughnuts through step 3 and freeze unbaked. Place doughnuts and doughnut holes on a baking sheet in a single layer and freeze. Transfer to a 1-gallon (3.8 L) freezer bag.

## 🍞 TO REHEAT

Let doughnuts and doughnut holes come to room temperature. Preheat oven to 250°F (120°C, or gas mark ½) and place doughnuts and doughnut holes on baking sheets. Place in oven to warm. While warming, make the maple glaze.

OVEN METHOD: To reheat unbaked doughnuts, preheat oven to 350°F (180°C, or gas mark 4) and place doughnuts and doughnut holes on a greased baking sheet. Bake for 15 minutes or until lightly browned and cooked through.

TO MAKE GLAZE: In a small saucepan, whisk together sugar, maple syrup, and water. Bring to a boil over medium-high heat and keep at a boil, stirring occasionally, for 4 to 5 minutes. Set aside to cool for 15 minutes. Stir in vanilla extract. Drizzle over doughnuts.

# SAVORY ZUCCHINI MUFFINS

If zucchini has overrun your garden, shred it and make these savory zucchini muffins, punctuated with herb, cheese, and walnut flavors, to pair delectably with salads, soups, stews, and roasted meats. For a tasty change, substitute shredded carrots for zucchini.

1 cup (125 g) all-purpose flour

1½ cups (180 g) whole-wheat pastry flour

4 teaspoons (18.4 g) baking powder

½ teaspoon salt

2 eggs

⅔ cup (160 ml) milk

⅓ cup (80 ml) extra-virgin olive oil

1 cup (120 g) shredded zucchini

1 clove garlic, minced

1 tablespoon (6 g) grated lemon zest

3 tablespoons (12 g) thyme leaves

1 tablespoon (3 g) minced chives

A few grinds black pepper

⅓ cup (33 g) freshly grated Parmesan cheese

½ cup (60g ) chopped toasted walnuts

① Preheat oven to 425°F (220°C, or gas mark 7). Grease a 12-cup muffin pan.

② In a large bowl, sift together flours, baking powder, and salt. In a second bowl, whisk together eggs, milk, and oil.

③ Add egg mixture to flour mixture and beat until just blended. Stir in zucchini, garlic, lemon zest, thyme, chives, pepper, cheese, and walnuts.

④ Fill muffin pan. Bake for 16 to 18 minutes or until muffins are just done. Cool in pan on a wire rack for 10 minutes. Remove from the pan and cool completely.

YIELD: 12 MUFFINS, OR 12 SERVINGS

##  TO FREEZE

Place muffins on a baking sheet and place in the freezer until solid. Wrap individually with freezer wrap or place muffins in a 1-gallon (3.8 L) freezer bag, removing as much air as possible before sealing.

## 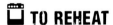 TO REHEAT

Thaw muffins at room temperature. To serve warm, place muffins back in muffin pan and reheat in a 350°F (180°C, or gas mark 4) oven.

## COOKING TIP: FREEZE ZUCCHINI

Whether you harvest your garden or stock up at the farmers' market, you can freeze zucchini so you have a taste of summer year-round. To freeze zucchini: Steam shredded zucchini for 2 to 3 minutes, dip in a cold water bath, drain, and freeze in freezer-safe bags or containers. After thawing, squeeze out excess moisture and toss in with hot pasta or rice, use in baked goods, or stir into ground meat fillings.

AMOUNT PER SERVING: Calories 216.59; Total Fat 11.42 g; Cholesterol 38.78 mg; Sodium 321.57 mg; Potassium 123.13 mg; Total Carbohydrates 23.02 g; Fiber 1.61 g; Sugar 1.2 g; Protein 6.26 g

# BANANA-COCONUT MUFFINS

A breakfast treat with tropical flair, banana and coconut turn ordinary morning muffins into something special. Bananas, a sweet source of vitamin B6 and potassium, keep muffins moist while coconut, rich in manganese and a good source of fiber, adds a toasty flavor and chewy texture. Unsweetened toasted coconut flakes are available at Trader Joe's; unsweetened coconut flakes are also available from Bob's Red Mill. You can toast coconut flakes in a dry skillet over medium heat.

**1 cup (125 g) all-purpose flour**

**1¼ cups (150 g) whole-wheat pastry flour**

**2 teaspoons baking powder**

**1 teaspoon baking soda**

**½ teaspoon salt**

**1½ teaspoons ground cinnamon**

**½ teaspoon ground allspice**

**¼ cup (55 g) unsalted butter, room temperature**

**¼ cup (60 g) Greek style plain yogurt**

**¼ cup (60 g) packed brown sugar**

**3 eggs**

**1 teaspoon pure vanilla extract**

**3 very ripe bananas, mashed (about 2 cups)**

**¾ cup (64 g) toasted coconut flakes**

① Preheat oven to 375°F (190°C, or gas mark 5) and generously spray a 12-cup muffin pan with nonstick cooking spray.

② In a medium bowl, whisk together flours, baking powder, baking soda, salt, cinnamon, and allspice. Set aside.

③ In the bowl of a standup mixer fitted with the paddle attachment, beat butter, yogurt, and sugar until well-combined. Beat in eggs one at a time and then add vanilla. Mix in bananas.

④ Add flour mixture and mix until just combined. Stir in coconut flakes.

⑤ Divide batter evenly in muffin cups. Bake for 15 minutes or until tops are just golden and muffins spring back when touched. Let cool in pan for 5 minutes and then invert onto a wire rack to cool completely.

YIELD: 12 MUFFINS, OR 12 SERVINGS

 **TO FREEZE**

Place muffins on a baking sheet and place in the freezer until solid. Wrap individually with freezer wrap or place muffins in a 1-gallon (3.8 L) freezer bag, removing as much air as possible before sealing.

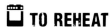 **TO REHEAT**

Thaw muffins at room temperature.

OVEN METHOD: To serve warm, place muffins back in muffin pan and reheat in a 350°F (180°C, or gas mark 4) oven.

AMOUNT PER SERVING: Calories 205.77; Total Fat 6.98 g; Cholesterol 63.04 mg; Sodium 322.3 mg; Potassium 226.53 mg; Total Carbohydrates 32.24 g; Fiber 3.25 g; Sugar 10.59 g; Protein 5.24 g

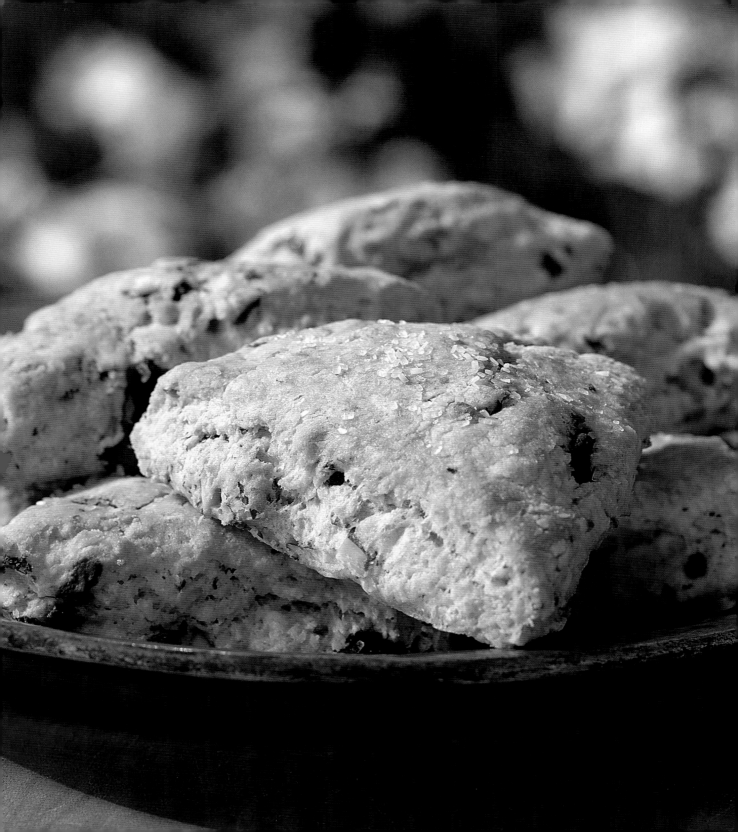

# DARK CHOCOLATE AND ALMOND SCONES

The heart-healthy and undeniably delicious combination of dark chocolate and almonds makes these scones an irresistible make-ahead breakfast food.

1 cup (125 g) all-purpose flour

1 cup (120 g) whole-wheat pastry flour

2½ teaspoons (11.5 g) baking powder

½ teaspoon baking soda

½ teaspoon salt

½ cup (112 g) unsalted butter, chilled, cubed

¾ cup (128 g) chopped 85% dark chocolate bar

¾ cup (75 g) chopped toasted almonds

2 eggs

½ cup (120 ml) evaporated milk

1 teaspoon pure almond extract

2 tablespoons (12 g) finely grated lemon zest

2 to 3 tablespoons (28 to 45 ml) milk

Raw or turbinado sugar

① Preheat oven to 425°F (220°C, or gas mark 7) and grease a large baking sheet.

② In a large bowl, whisk together flours, baking powder, baking soda, and salt. Use a pastry cutter or your fingers to cut butter into flour mixture until it resembles a coarse meal. Add chocolate and almonds, tossing to combine.

③ In a small bowl, whisk together eggs, evaporated milk, almond extract, and lemon zest. Add to flour mixture, stirring until just combined and moist. Turn dough out onto a lightly floured surface and use your hands to bring dough together into a ball.

④ Divide dough in half and pat each portion into a ½-inch (1.3 cm) -thick disk. Using a sharp floured knife, cut each disk into 6 pie-shaped pieces. Brush excess flour from the scones and arrange them on the prepared baking sheet.

⑤ Using a pastry brush, brush scones with milk and sprinkle with sugar. Bake for 12 minutes or until just golden. Transfer to wire racks to cool completely.

YIELD: 12 SCONES, OR 12 SERVINGS

## SERVING SUGGESTIONS

Dark Chocolate and Almond Scones can do double duty as a dynamite dessert. Split scones and fill with fresh strawberries and unsweetened whipped cream or Greek yogurt for an indulgent twist on strawberry shortcake or crumble a scone on top of a scoop of vanilla or chocolate ice cream.

 ## TO FREEZE

Place scones on a baking sheet and freeze until solid. Tightly wrap individual scones in freezer wrap or place multiple scones in 1-gallon (3.8 L) freezer-safe bags.

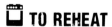 ## TO REHEAT

Let scones come to room temperature.

OVEN METHOD: Preheat oven to 350°F (180°C, or gas mark 4). Place scones on a baking sheet and warm in oven for 5 to 8 minutes or until heated through.

AMOUNT PER SERVING: Calories 265.09; Total Fat 18.92 g; Cholesterol 58.61 mg; Sodium 279.42 mg; Potassium 246.84 mg; Total Carbohydrates 21.78 g; Fiber 4.29 g; Sugar 1.82 g; Protein 7.39 g

# CHAPTER 11

## DESSERTS

### SWEET SELECTIONS THAT ARE WHOLESOME TO BOOT

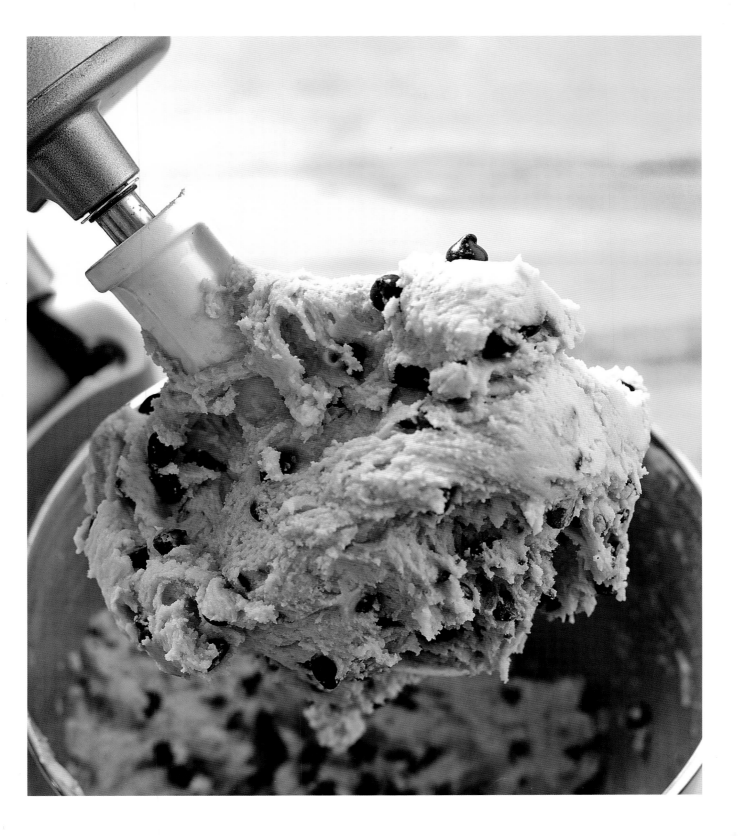

# DOUBLE-CRUST WHOLE-WHEAT PIE DOUGH

Keeping pie dough on hand gives you nearly endless culinary possibilities. This whole-grain pie dough can be used for dessert pies and tarts, or you can omit the sugar and use it for quiche, appetizers, or savory turnovers.

1½ cups (188 g) all-purpose flour

1½ cups (180 g) whole-wheat pastry flour

3 tablespoons (39 g) granulated sugar

1 teaspoon salt

1 cup (225 g) unsalted butter, chilled, cut into small pieces

¼ cup (50 g) vegetable shortening, chilled, cut into small pieces

⅓ to ½ cup (80 to 120 ml) iced water

① Place flours, sugar, and salt in a food processor and pulse to combine. Add butter and shortening and pulse to cut into flour until a coarse meal forms.

② Add ⅓ cup (80 ml) water and pulse until dough starts to come together. If dough seems dry, add a bit more water. Dump dough onto a lightly floured surface or pastry mat and gently knead dough into a ball. Divide the dough into 2 parts. Flatten each part into a disk.

YIELD: 2 PIE CRUSTS, OR 16 SERVINGS
(8 SERVINGS IF MAKING ONE DOUBLE-CRUST PIE)

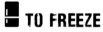 **TO FREEZE**

Wrap each disk tightly in plastic wrap or freezer wrap and place in a 1-gallon (3.8 L) freezer bag.

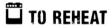 **TO REHEAT**

Place dough in refrigerator to thaw for a few hours. Roll it out and use according to recipe directions.

AMOUNT PER SERVING:  Calories 223.93; Total Fat 14.76 g; Cholesterol 31.98 mg; Sodium 147.36 mg; Potassium 28.6 mg; Total Carbohydrates 20.38 g; Fiber 0.63 g; Sugar 2.51 g; Protein 2.55 g

# IMPRESS-THE-GUESTS PEACH PIE

Spicy peaches nestled in a whole-grain pie crust is the quintessential summer dessert. Serve this pie at your next cookout or bake it as a sweet surprise for your family when peach season has long passed.

...................................................................................................................................................................

**1 recipe Double Crust Whole-Wheat Pie Dough (page 204)**

**5 cups (850 g) fresh ripe peach slices, peeled**

**½ cup (115 g) firmly packed brown sugar**

**¼ cup (50 g) granulated sugar**

**½ cup (63 g) all-purpose flour**

**1 teaspoon ground cinnamon**

**½ teaspoon freshly grated nutmeg**

**Pinch of ground cloves**

**2 tablespoons (28 ml) lemon juice**

**1 tablespoon (6 g) finely grated lemon zest**

① Roll out bottom pie crust to fit in a 9 (23 cm) pie plate with 1-inch (2.5 cm) overhang. Line pie plate with crust. Roll out top crust to fit over top pie plate with 1½ inches (3.8 cm) overhang. Set top crust aside covered with a towel.

② In a large bowl, toss together peaches, sugars, flour, cinnamon, nutmeg, cloves, lemon juice, and lemon zest. Pour into pie plate. Place top crust over pie and fold the edges of the top crust over and under the bottom edges and flute with your fingertips to seal. You can also seal edges with the tines of a fork.

YIELD: 1 PIE, OR 8 SERVINGS

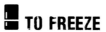 **TO FREEZE**

Place pie in freezer until firm. Cover tightly with aluminum foil.

 **TO BAKE**

OVEN METHOD: Preheat oven to 425°F (220°C, or gas mark 7). Remove foil and cut a few slits in top crust to vent. Bake for 15 minutes and then reduce heat to 350°F (180°C, or gas mark 4). Bake for 45 minutes or until crust is golden and peaches are bubbly. If the crust edges start to brown too quickly, place a piece of aluminum foil around the rim. Let cool on a wire rack for at least 20 minutes before slicing and serving.

AMOUNT PER SERVING: Calories 559.55; Total Fat 29.92 g; Cholesterol 63.97 mg; Sodium 299.04 mg; Potassium 294.3 mg; Total Carbohydrates 78.01 g; Fiber 3.37 g; Sugar 34.31 g; Protein 6.94 g

# QUICK APRICOT-WALNUT COBBLER

Juicy apricots are a natural for a tender cobbler topping. The addition of lime, ginger, and cumin give this dessert a unique flavor profile that makes it an extra-special dessert. Pair cobbler with a small scoop of vanilla ice cream or top it with a dollop of honey-flavored Greek yogurt.

**2½ pounds (1.1 kg) ripe apricots, pitted, sliced**

**2 tablespoons (26 g) granulated sugar**

**1 tablespoon (8 g) all-purpose flour**

**Juice of 1 lime**

**1 cup (120 g) whole-wheat pastry flour**

**⅔ cup (150 g) packed brown sugar**

**½ cup (112 g) unsalted butter, cut into small pieces**

**½ cup (60 g) coarsely chopped walnuts**

**1 teaspoon ground cinnamon**

**½ teaspoon ground ginger**

**½ teaspoon ground cumin**

① In a large mixing bowl, combine apricots, granulated sugar, all-purpose flour, and lime juice, tossing to combine. Pour into a 9-inch (23 cm) square baking dish or aluminum baking pan.

② In a food processor, combine pastry flour, brown sugar, butter, walnuts, cinnamon, ginger, and cumin. Pulse to combine until crumbly. Sprinkle crumb topping over apricot mixture.

YIELD: ONE 9-INCH (23 CM) COBBLER, OR 8 SERVINGS

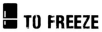 **TO FREEZE**

Lay a piece of plastic wrap directly on topping. Tightly wrap with aluminum foil.

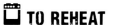 **TO REHEAT**

Preheat oven to 375°F (190°C, or gas mark 5). Remove wrap and foil. Place frozen cobbler in oven and bake for 1 hour or until topping is toasted and apricot mixture is bubbly.

AMOUNT PER SERVING: Calories 336.95; Total Fat 16.78 g; Cholesterol 30.1 mg; Sodium 8.47 mg; Potassium 308.27 mg; Total Carbohydrates 45.49 g; Fiber 2.86 g; Sugar 29.62 g; Protein 4.25 g

# LIGHT AND LUSCIOUS BLUEBERRY CHEESECAKE

A classic dessert, blueberry cheesecake is given a low-carb makeover by replacing graham crackers with almond flour for the crust and using a minimum amount of sugar for sweetness. You can find almond flour in the bulk section of natural food stores as well as the baking aisle of many supermarkets. Almond meal can be used but will have a denser texture.

⅓ **cup (75 g) unsalted butter, melted, divided**

**2 cups (230 g) almond flour**

**2 cups (460 g) cream cheese, softened at room temperature**

**1 cup (250 g) ricotta cheese**

**Juice and grated zest of 1 lemon**

**5 eggs**

**¼ to ½ cup (50 to 100 g) granulated sugar**

**2 teaspoons pure vanilla extract**

**2 cups blueberries, (290 g) fresh or (310 g) frozen**

① Preheat oven to 425°F (220°C, or gas mark 7). Grease a 9-inch (23 cm) springform pan with 1 tablespoon (14 g) butter.

② In a medium bowl, mix almond flour with remaining butter. Spread the mixture on the bottom of the prepared pan and smooth the top. Bake for 10 minutes or until lightly browned.

③ Remove the pan from the oven and allow to cool on a wire rack. Reduce the heat of the oven to 350°F (180°C, or gas mark 4).

④ In the bowl of a standup mixer fitted with the paddle attachment, beat the cheeses, lemon juice and zest, and eggs together in a large bowl until smooth. Add sugar and vanilla, beating until smooth. Fold in blueberries.

⑤ Wrap bottom and sides of springform pan with foil. Pour batter into springform pan and smooth top with a spatula.

⑥ Place springform pan in a large, deep baking dish and pour boiling water into baking dish until it is half full. Bake for 1 hour. Check cheesecake. If it is just set and no longer liquidy, remove from oven. If it is still jiggly with liquid, bake for 10 minutes or until the top sets. Do not overcook to the point that the cheesecake dries out and cracks.

⑦ Remove cheesecake from water bath and cool on a wire rack. Remove foil and refrigerate for a few hours or overnight to cool completely. Run a dull knife or thin spatula in between the cake and the sides of the pan. Loosen and remove sides of pan.

YIELD: 16 SERVINGS

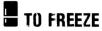 **TO FREEZE**

Place cheesecake in freezer for 1 hour. Wrap cake with plastic wrap and then heavy-duty aluminum foil.

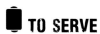 **TO SERVE**

Thaw cheesecake in refrigerator overnight.

AMOUNT PER SERVING: Calories 563.2; Total Fat 47.95 g; Cholesterol 112.64 mg; Sodium 127.54 mg; Potassium 101.89 mg; Total Carbohydrates 21.75 g; Fiber 7.45 g; Sugar 7.58 g; Protein 19.56 g

# DECADENT DARK CHOCOLATE MINT CAKE

Chocolate and mint are an unbeatable pair in this indulgently moist cake. Serve modest slices with a small scoop of reduced-fat vanilla ice cream. Whole-wheat pastry flour is a wholesome substitute for all-purpose flour. If you want to make a frosted layer cake, do not reheat. Simply thaw and frost.

1½ cups (255 g) chopped dark chocolate

½ cup (or 112 g) butter, softened at room temperature

1 cup (225 g) firmly packed brown sugar

1 cup (200 g) mint sugar*

3 large eggs

2 cups (240 g) whole-wheat pastry flour

1 teaspoon baking soda

½ teaspoon salt

1 container (8 ounces, or 225 g) plain whole-milk yogurt

1 cup (235 ml) hot water

1½ teaspoons pure vanilla extract

½ teaspoon mint extract

① Preheat oven to 350°F (180°C, or gas mark 4). Grease and flour two 10-inch (25 cm) cake pans.

② In a double boiler, melt chocolate, stirring often, until smooth.

③ In a standup mixer fitted with the paddle attachment, beat butter and sugars at medium speed until well-blended. Add eggs, 1 at a time, beating just until blended after each addition. Slowly add melted chocolate, beating just until blended.

④ Sift together flour, baking soda, and salt in a medium bowl. Gradually add flour mixture to chocolate mixture alternately with yogurt, beginning and ending with flour mixture. Beat at low speed just until blended after each addition.

⑤ Gradually add 1 cup (235 ml) hot water in a slow, steady stream, beating at low speed just until blended. Stir in vanilla and mint. Spoon batter evenly into prepared cake pans.

⑥ Bake for 30 minutes or until a wooden pick inserted in center of cake comes out clean. Cool in pans on a wire rack for 10 minutes, remove from pans, and let cool completely on wire rack.

YIELD: TWO 10-INCH (25 CM) CAKES, OR 16 SERVINGS

*Note: To make mint sugar, lightly crush a handful of fresh mint leaves and place them in a bowl. Add granulated sugar and toss to combine. Cover tightly and let sugar sit for 1 week. Remove mint leaves before using.

## NUTRITION SPOTLIGHT: DARK CHOCOLATE

Though dark chocolate is considered one of the most decadent of sweets, it is also the healthiest. It is chock-full of flavonoids, phytonutrients that have potent antioxidant power, and the combination of fat and sugar in chocolate can raise serotonin and endorphins in the brain. The key is consuming modest amounts so you don't overdo on the calories. The darker the chocolate the better. Reach for dark chocolate bars that are at least 85% cocoa.

AMOUNT PER SERVING: Calories 314.48; Total Fat 15.82 g; Cholesterol 56.55 mg; Sodium 179.98 mg; Potassium 208.96 mg; Total Carbohydrates 43.91 g; Fiber 3.15 g; Sugar 27.11 g; Protein 5.48 g

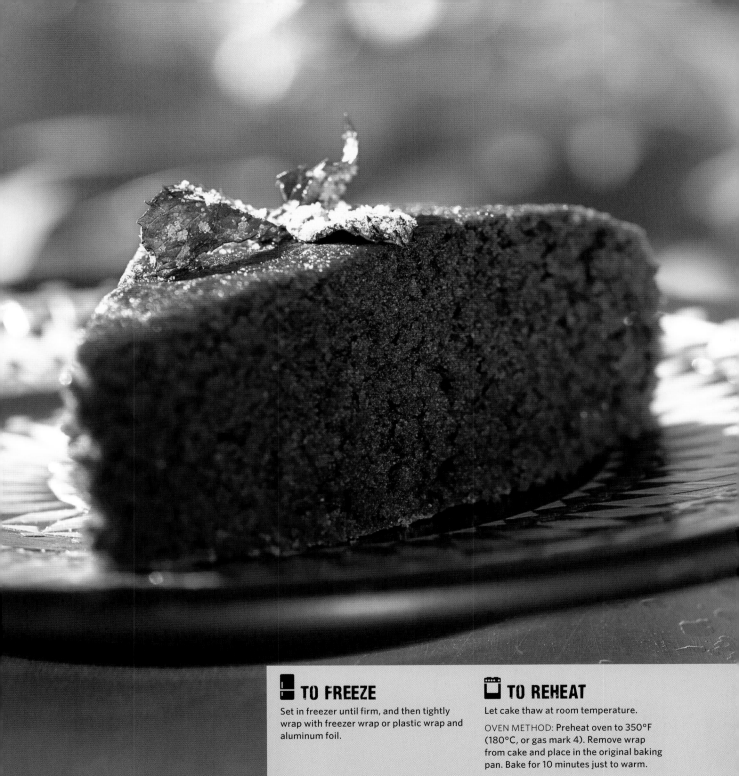

## 🧊 TO FREEZE

Set in freezer until firm, and then tightly wrap with freezer wrap or plastic wrap and aluminum foil.

## 🔲 TO REHEAT

Let cake thaw at room temperature.

OVEN METHOD: Preheat oven to 350°F (180°C, or gas mark 4). Remove wrap from cake and place in the original baking pan. Bake for 10 minutes just to warm.

# BLACKBERRY BUTTERMILK CAKE

Blackberries lend their nutrient-dense deliciousness in this cake while the buttermilk gives it a lovely moistness. Apricot preserves not only steps in for sugar, it adds an additional nuance of fruit flavor.

........................................................................................................................................................................

**1½ cups (180 g) whole-wheat pastry flour**

**2 tablespoons (14 g) ground flaxseed**

**1 teaspoon salt**

**1 teaspoon baking powder**

**½ teaspoon baking soda**

**½ cup (112 g) unsalted butter**

**1 cup (320 g) apricot preserves**

**2 teaspoons vanilla extract**

**1 egg**

**1 cup (235 ml) buttermilk**

**1 pint (290 g) blackberries**

**2 tablespoons (26 g) raw or turbinado sugar**

① Preheat oven to 350°F (180°C, or gas mark 4). Butter and flour a 9-inch (23 cm) springform pan.

② In a large bowl, sift together flour, ground flax, salt, baking powder, and baking soda. Set aside.

③ In a second large bowl, beat butter and preserves until well-combined. Beat in vanilla and egg. Add buttermilk and flour mixture, alternating two or three times, mixing until just combined and moistened.

④ Pour batter into prepared springform pan. Scatter blackberries over the batter and then sprinkle with raw sugar.

⑤ Bake for 40 minutes or until a cake tester inserted in the center comes out dry. Let cake cool in the pan on a wire rack for 10 to 15 minutes and then release the sides and allow cake to cool completely.

YIELD: ONE 9-INCH (23 CM) CAKE, OR 8 SERVINGS

## COOKING TIP: LEARN THE BENEFITS OF BUTTERMILK

Despite the word "butter" as part of its name, buttermilk is a healthy substitute for many higher-fat dairy ingredients. Here are some suggestions:

- Use in place of butter or milk (or both) in mashed potatoes.
- Substitute for part of the cream or sour cream in sweet or savory recipes.
- Make smoothies by using buttermilk in place of regular milk or yogurt.
- Add to pancakes, waffles, muffins, scones, cakes, and quick breads instead of milk or cream.
- Replace part of the milk or cream with buttermilk in creamy soups.

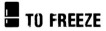 **TO FREEZE**

Wrap completely cooled cake tightly in freezer wrap or in plastic wrap and a sheet of aluminum foil.

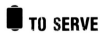 **TO SERVE**

Allow cake to thaw at room temperature.

AMOUNT PER SERVING: Calories 347.02; Total Fat 13.34 g; Cholesterol 57.75 mg; Sodium 490.03 mg; Potassium 181.23 mg; Total Carbohydrates 52.44 g; Fiber 2.82 g; Sugar 24.12 g; Protein 5.33 g

# LOW-FAT CHOCOLATE CHERRY BROWNIES

Chocolate brownies get a healthy makeover with a low-fat brownie mix and the addition of antioxidant-rich cherries. Tuck these yummy brownies in your kids' lunch bag for a sweet treat that will brighten up their school day.

**1 package (20.5 ounces, or 575 g) low-fat fudge brownie mix**

**½ cup (115 g) plain whole-milk yogurt**

**1 egg, lightly beaten**

**1 cup (320 g) cherry preserves**

① Preheat oven to 350°F (180°C, or gas mark 4). Grease a 13 x 9-inch (33 x 23 cm) baking dish.

② Mix together brownie mix, yogurt, and egg until well-combined and smooth. Pour into the prepared baking dish.

③ Using a spoon, drop cherry jam onto brownie batter. Use a dull knife to cut jam through batter. Bake for 25 minutes or according to package directions. A knife inserted 2 inches (5 cm) from the side should come out clean.

④ Let cool in the pan for 15 minutes and then invert onto a plate and onto a wire rack to cool completely.

YIELD: 18 BROWNIES, OR 18 SERVINGS

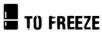 **TO FREEZE**

INDIVIDUAL SERVINGS: Cut into 18 brownies and tightly wrap each one with freezer wrap or plastic wrap. Place in a 1-gallon (3.8 L) freezer bag.

FOR A CROWD: Place large brownie onto a baking sheet and freeze until firm. Tightly wrap with freezer wrap or plastic wrap and heavy-duty aluminum foil.

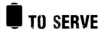 **TO SERVE**

Thaw brownies at room temperature until soft. Remove wrapping after thawed.

MICROWAVE METHOD: To serve warm, microwave individual brownies on high for 30 seconds or until heated through.

OVEN METHOD: Preheat oven to 350°F (180°C, or gas mark 4). Place large brownie in original baking dish and reheat for 10 minutes or until heated through.

AMOUNT PER SERVING: Calories 101.67; Total Fat 1.24 g; Cholesterol 12.14 mg; Sodium 53.19 mg; Potassium 32.35 mg; Total Carbohydrates 21.9 g; Fiber 0.54 g; Sugar 14.77 g; Protein 1.43 g

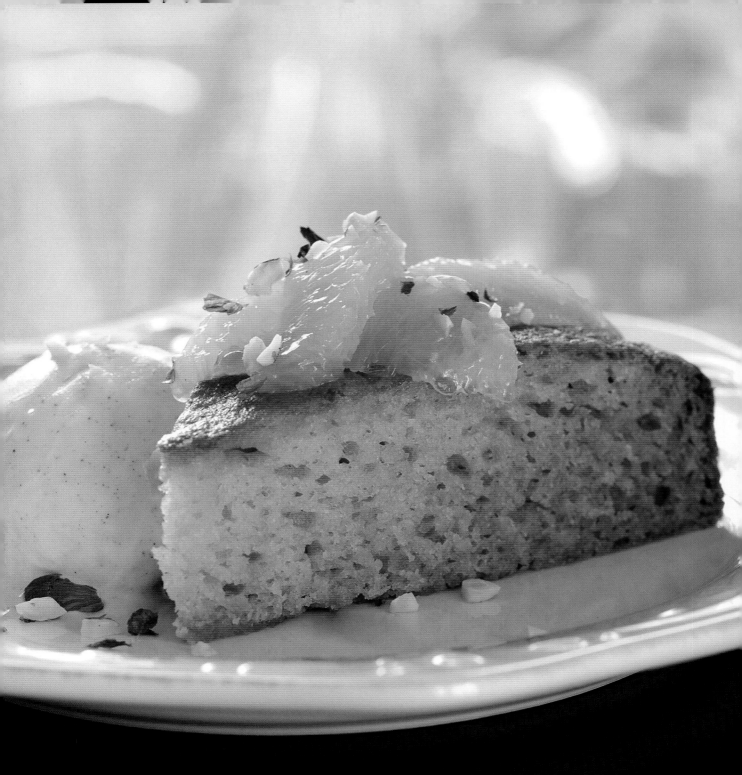

_Try_ *

# CITRUS-FLAVORED OLIVE OIL CAKE

An Italian-inspired dessert made with olive oil, this honey orange cake is a heart-healthy alternative to cakes made with butter and loads of sugar. For a seasonal change, substitute blood oranges for regular oranges during winter and early spring.

**Juice of 2 oranges (about ⅔ cup, or 160 ml)**

**½ cup (170 g) warmed honey**

**¼ cup (60 ml) extra-virgin olive oil**

**2 large eggs, separated**

**2 tablespoons (12 g) finely grated orange zest**

**1⅔ cups (208 g) all-purpose flour, sifted**

**½ cup (100 g) granulated sugar**

**1 teaspoon baking powder**

**½ teaspoon baking soda**

① Preheat oven to 350°F (180°C, or gas mark 4). Lightly grease and flour bottom and sides of a 9-inch (23 cm) springform pan. Set aside.

② In a standup mixer fitted with the paddle attachment, mix orange juice, honey, olive oil, egg yolks, and orange zest on medium speed until well-blended.

③ In a medium bowl, whisk together flour, sugar, baking powder, and baking soda. In a small bowl, beat egg whites until soft peaks form.

④ With mixer on low speed, add flour mixture to orange juice mixture, blending until just moistened. With a spatula, gently fold in egg whites. Pour batter into prepared pan.

⑤ Bake for 35 minutes or until a cake tester inserted in the center comes out clean. Cool 10 minutes on a wire rack and then remove sides from pan and cool completely. Just before serving, sprinkle with confectioners' sugar.

YIELD: ONE 9-INCH (23 CM) CAKE, OR 8 SERVINGS

## SERVING SUGGESTION

Pair Citrus-Flavored Olive Oil Cake with a vanilla or hazelnut gelato for the full Italian dessert experience. Garnish with chopped toasted hazelnuts and orange slices for a brilliant contrast in color. Cake can also be cubed and transformed into a trifle any time of year.

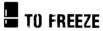 **TO FREEZE**

Tightly wrap cake in freezer wrap or in plastic wrap and a sheet of aluminum foil.

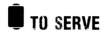 **TO SERVE**

Let cake thaw in refrigerator. Serve dusted with confectioners' sugar and garnished with orange slices and a dollop of plain whole-milk yogurt.

AMOUNT PER SERVING: Calories 297.21; Total Fat 8.39 g; Cholesterol 52.88 mg; Sodium 158.87 mg; Potassium 101.16 mg; Total Carbohydrates 52.66 g; Fiber 0.95 g; Sugar 31.87 g; Protein 4.49 g

# DARK CHOCOLATE CHIP COOKIE DOUGH

Decadent chunks of dark chocolate nestled in a whole-grain cookie make this dessert hard to resist. Keeping a few logs in your freezer means ready-to-bake cookies in minutes without the flour mess on the counter or the doughy bowls in the sink.

2 cups (400 g) vegetable shortening

1 cup (200 g) granulated sugar

1¾ cups (395 g) firmly packed brown sugar

4 eggs

2 teaspoons pure vanilla extract

3 cups (375 g) all-purpose flour

2 cups (240 g) whole-wheat pastry flour

2 teaspoons (9 g) baking soda

2 teaspoons salt

3 bars (3.5 ounces, or 100 g, each) 85% dark chocolate bars, chopped

① In the bowl of a standup mixer fitted with the paddle attachment, beat shortening and sugars until well-combined. Beat in eggs, one at a time, until incorporated. Beat in vanilla.

② In a second large bowl, whisk together flours, baking soda, and salt. Add flour mixture to shortening mixture and blend until a dough forms, scraping down sides of the bowl occasionally. Add chocolate, blending until just combined. Divide dough into 4 even parts and roll each part into a log.

YIELD: 10 DOZEN COOKIES (30 COOKIES PER LOG), OR 120 SERVINGS

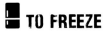 TO FREEZE

Tightly wrap each log in plastic wrap. Place in a 1-gallon (3.8 L) freezer bag and freeze for up to 6 months.

 TO BAKE

OVEN METHOD: Preheat oven to 350°F (180°C, or gas mark 4). Let cookie dough thaw at room temperature for 10 to 15 minutes while the oven is preheating. Use a sharp knife to slice logs crosswise into cookies. Place on large baking sheets and bake for 10 to 12 minutes or until cookies are set. Let cool on baking sheets for 5 minutes then transfer to wire racks to cool.

NOTE: Cookies can be baked before freezing. Bake until just done, let cool completely, freeze on a baking sheet, and transfer frozen cookies to freezer bags, removing as much air as possible before sealing. Thaw at room temperature.

AMOUNT PER SERVING: Calories 82.77; Total Fat 4.29 g; Cholesterol 8.92 mg; Sodium 62.93 mg; Potassium 12.53 mg; Total Carbohydrates 10.48 g; Fiber 0.29 g; Sugar 4.91 g; Protein 0.86 g

# OATMEAL-CINNAMON COOKIES

The scent of oatmeal cinnamon cookies is enough to bring the family running to the oven. Keeping a ready supply in your freezer will mean you can lure them to lunch or dinner in mere minutes—simply reheat in your oven for an intoxicating waft of oat cookie goodness.

1 cup (120 g) whole-wheat flour

1 cup (125 g) all-purpose flour

2 teaspoons baking powder

½ teaspoon ground cinnamon

¼ teaspoon freshly ground nutmeg

1 teaspoon salt

⅔ cup (160 ml) vegetable oil

1 cup (225 g) firmly packed brown sugar

2 eggs

2 teaspoons pure vanilla extract

1 cup (80 g) rolled oats

1½ cups (263 g) cinnamon chips

① Preheat oven to 350°F (180°C, or gas mark 4) and line 2 baking sheets with parchment paper. In a large bowl, whisk together flours, baking powder, cinnamon, nutmeg, and salt.

② In the bowl of a standup mixer fitted with the paddle attachment, beat oil and brown sugar together. Add eggs, one at a time, beating until smooth. Beat in vanilla.

③ Add flour mixture to egg mixture and blend on low until just moist. Add oats and cinnamon chips, blending on low until just combined.

④ Using 2 tablespoonfuls (28 g) per cookie, roll dough into balls and set them on prepared baking sheets 1 to 2 inches (2.5 to 5 cm) apart. Bake for 8 minutes, rotate sheets, and bake for 5 minutes more or until cookies are just lightly browned.

⑤ Let cool on sheets for a few minutes and then transfer to wire racks to cool completely.

YIELD: 36 COOKIES, OR 36 SERVINGS

## NUTRITION TIP: EAT OATS FOR HEART HEALTH

Here's how to up your oat intake and improve your health by:

- Eating a bowl of oatmeal for breakfast
- Making Oat-Rageous Cinnamon Brown Sugar Waffles (page 181)
- Adding oats to muffins, breads, or other baked goods
- Grinding rolled oats into flour and replacing part of the all-purpose flour in recipes
- Mixing rolled oats into the topping for fruit crumbles and crisps

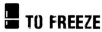 TO FREEZE

Place cookies on a baking sheet and freeze until solid. Transfer to a freezer container, stacking with a layer of waxed or parchment paper in between.

 TO SERVE

Let cookies thaw at room temperature for 1 to 2 hours.

OVEN METHOD: To serve warm, preheat oven to 350°F (180°C, or gas mark 4). Place cookies on a baking sheet and bake for 4 to 5 minutes or until warmed through.

AMOUNT PER SERVING: Calories 137.82; Total Fat 6.4 g; Cholesterol 11.75 mg; Sodium 111.73 mg; Potassium 39.19 mg; Total Carbohydrates 18.47 g; Fiber 1 g; Sugar 9.32 g; Protein 1.49 g

# DRIED BLUEBERRY AND COCONUT OAT BARS

Dried blueberries are concentrated gems of antioxidants that add color and texture to these whole-grain dessert bars. Brown rice syrup, a natural sweetener, eliminates the need for sugar, and shredded coconut offers a tropical dose of fiber and healthy fats.

2 eggs

½ cup (115 g) packed brown sugar

¼ cup (85 g) brown rice syrup

3 tablespoons (45 ml) canola oil

2 teaspoons pure vanilla extract

1 cup (120 g) whole-wheat pastry flour

½ cup (63 g) all-purpose flour

1 teaspoon baking soda

½ teaspoon salt

1 teaspoon ground cinnamon

½ teaspoon ground allspice

1½ cups (120 g) rolled oats

½ cup (60 g) dried blueberries

½ cup (43 g) unsweetened shredded coconut

① Preheat oven to 350°F (180°C, or gas mark 4). Grease a 13 x 9-inch (33 x 23 cm) baking dish.

② In the bowl of a standup mixer fitted with the paddle attachment, mix eggs, brown sugar, and brown rice syrup until smooth. Add oil and vanilla and blend until smooth.

③ In a medium bowl, whisk together flours, baking soda, salt, cinnamon, allspice, and oats. Add to egg mixture and blend on low speed until moist. Blend in blueberries and coconut.

④ Transfer to prepared baking dish and press into pan. Bake for 25 to 30 minutes or until lightly browned. Let cool for 10 minutes. Invert onto a wire rack to cool completely.

YIELD 12 TO 16 BARS, OR 12 TO 16 SERVINGS

## NUTRITION SPOTLIGHT: BROWN RICE SYRUP IS SWEET

A mildly sweet, amber-colored liquid sweetener similar to honey, brown rice syrup is made from a nutritive sweetener that has a lower glycemic index value and is about half as sweet as sugar. Brown rice syrup is considered to be one of the healthiest sweeteners since it is produced from a whole food source, but it is still has calories and should be used in moderation like all sweeteners.

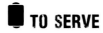

## TO FREEZE

INDIVIDUAL SERVINGS: Cut into 12 to 16 bars and wrap each with freezer wrap.

FOR A CROWD: Cut into 12 to 16 bars and place on a baking sheet. Freeze until solid. Transfer to a large freezer bag.

## TO SERVE

Let bars thaw at room temperature.

AMOUNT PER SERVING: Calories 171; Total Fat 5.52 g; Cholesterol 26.44 mg; Sodium 164.18 mg; Potassium 101.01 mg; Total Carbohydrates 22.35 g; Fiber 2.41 g; Sugar 7.89 g; Protein 3.47 g

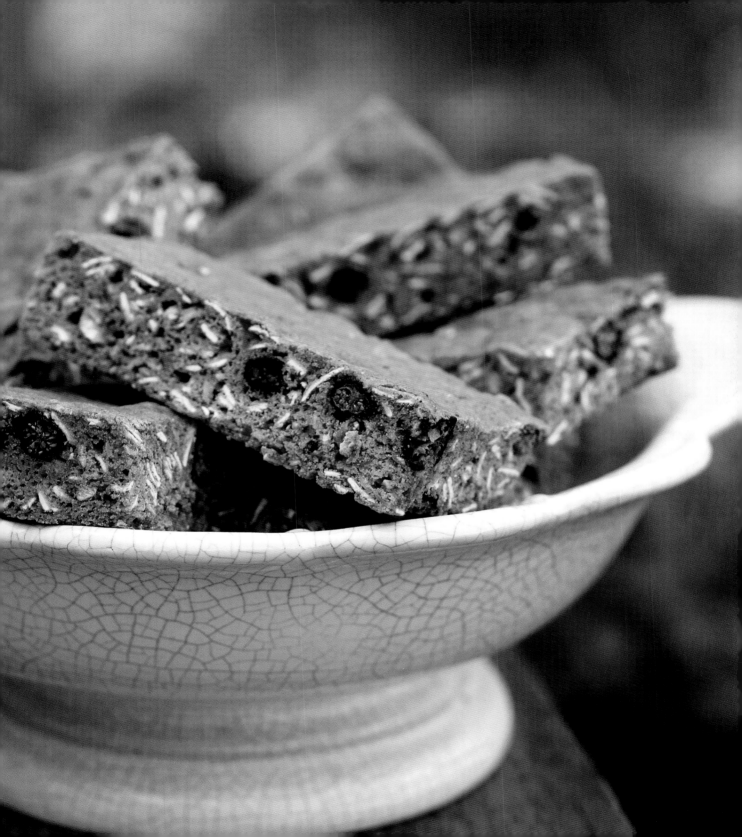

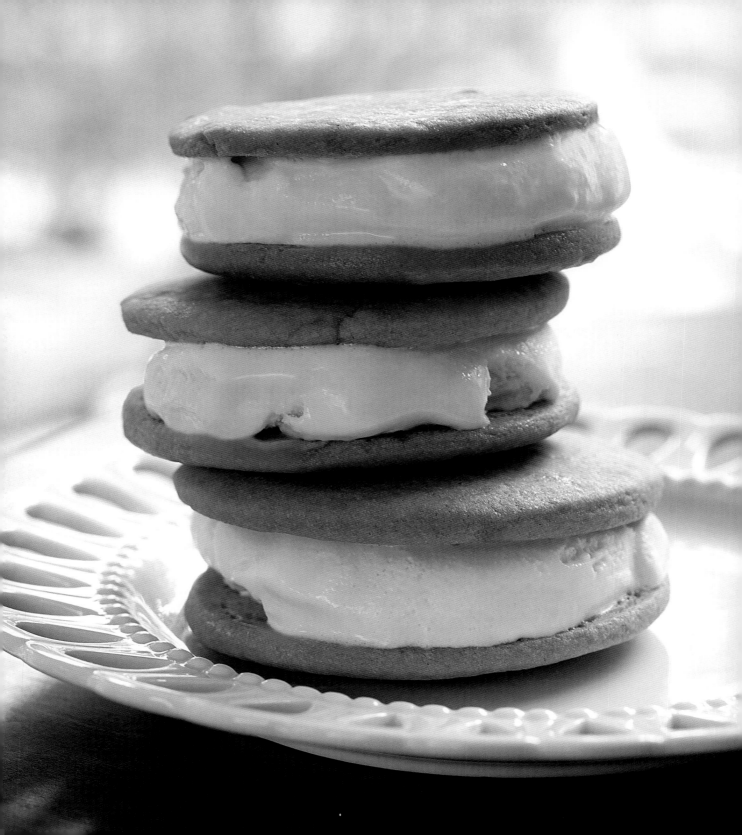

# ANYTIME LEMON COOKIE ICE CREAM SANDWICHES

Ice cream sandwiches evoke childhood nostalgia for adults and are quick palate-pleasers for kids. Sure, you can buy the usual chocolate cookie vanilla ice cream varieties at the supermarket, or you can make zesty batches of these lemon vanilla sandwiches and sink your sweet tooth into a homemade treat.

¾ cup (165 g) unsalted butter, softened

½ cup (115 g) firmly packed brown sugar

½ cup (100 g) granulated sugar

1 large egg

Finely grated zest of 1 lemon

1 teaspoon pure vanilla extract

2 cups (250 g) all-purpose flour

1 teaspoon baking powder

1 teaspoon baking soda

½ teaspoon salt

2 pints (570 g) reduced-fat vanilla ice cream, softened

① In a standup mixer fitted with the paddle attachment, beat butter and sugars until light and fluffy. Beat in the egg, lemon zest, and vanilla until well-combined.

② In a small bowl, whisk together flour, baking powder, baking soda, and salt. Add to mixer and blend until a sticky dough forms.

③ Remove dough from bowl and divide in half. On a sheet of parchment paper or waxed paper, roll each dough half into a log about 2 inches (5 cm) in diameter. Tightly wrap each log in the paper and refrigerate for 2 hours or until dough feels firm.

④ Preheat oven to 325°F (170°C, or gas mark 3). Line 2 baking sheets with parchment paper. Unwrap dough and slice each log into 15 rounds. Arrange on baking sheets.

⑤ Bake for 11 minutes or until the cookies are golden. Carefully transfer cookies to wire racks and cool completely.

⑥ When cookies are cool, spread a thick even layer of ice cream on half of the cookies. Place the second half of the cookies on top. Wrap each cookie tightly with plastic wrap and place in the freezer until firm.

YIELD: 15 ICE CREAM SANDWICHES, OR 15 SERVINGS

## COOKING TIP: SWAP CITRUS FOR CITRUS

In addition to being zesty high sources of vitamin C and other health-promoting phytonutrients, all varieties of citrus are bursting with a distinctive and refreshing flavor. Depending on the citrus that is in season or the fruit you have on hand, you can swap citrus for citrus for a change in your everyday recipes. For example, instead of using lemon here, substitute lime, orange, or tangerine.

AMOUNT PER SERVING: Calories 302.68; Total Fat 12.64 g; Cholesterol 54.83 mg; Sodium 247.22 mg; Potassium 171.64 mg; Total Carbohydrates 43.1 g; Fiber 0.97 g; Sugar 27.27 g; Protein 5.22 g

# FROZEN GINGER AND CHERRY COSMOS

Who says kids are the only ones who can enjoy a frozen ice pop? These ginger cherry pops are an adults-only treat that are fun to serve as an alternative to a mixed drink. Particularly fitting for summer poolside parties, frozen cosmos are a tasty way to take the taste of summer into the rest of the year.

**2¾ cups (650 ml) 100% cherry juice**

**1½ ounces (45 ml) SKYY Infusions Ginger Vodka**

**Juice of 1 small lime**

**6 pitted fresh cherries**

① Combine cherry juice, vodka, and lime juice in a large measuring glass with a pour spout. Place a cherry in each ice pop mold.

② Pour juice mixture into 6 ice pop molds. Place lids on molds or insert wooden ice pop sticks and freeze for 3 hours or until frozen.

YIELD: 6 FROZEN COSMOS, OR 16 SERVINGS

---

**NUTRITION SPOTLIGHT: CHERRIES**

A handful of fresh, frozen, or dried cherries a day or a glass of 100% cherry juice is a tasty way to sweeten up your heart health, combat cancer and diabetes, alleviate pain, promote sound sleep, and aid in muscle repair. In addition to the anti-inflammatory properties derived from their high level of antioxidants, cherries also contain melatonin, which has been found to help regulate the body's natural sleep patterns, prevent jet lag, reduce memory loss, and delay the aging process.

---

AMOUNT PER SERVING: Calories 87.57; Total Fat 0.04 g; Cholesterol 0 mg; Sodium 5.42 mg; Potassium 29.59 mg; Total Carbohydrates 16 g; Fiber 0.48 g; Sugar 11.63 g; Protein 0.27 g

# PERFECT PINEAPPLE-GINGER UPSIDE-DOWN CAKE

A cool and tropical take on pineapple upside-down cake, this frozen dessert is an impressive summer dinner party finale. Make an extra and keep it in your freezer for unexpected visitors or to surprise your family with a special sweet.

**8 ounces (225 g) angel food cake***

**1 can (20 ounces, or 570 g) pineapple rings packed in juice, drained, juice reserved**

**5 fresh sweet cherries, pitted**

**2 tablespoons (16 g) grated fresh ginger**

**½ teaspoon ground cinnamon**

**1 teaspoon pure vanilla extract**

**3 large egg yolks, at room temperature**

**¼ cup (60 g) firmly packed brown sugar**

**2 large egg whites, at room temperature**

**⅓ cup (67 g) granulated sugar**

**½ teaspoon cream of tartar**

**½ cup (120 ml) heavy cream**

> *Note: Place angel food cake in the freezer while preparing the rest of the ingredients. This will make it easier to slice. Do not freeze solid.

① Coat a 9-inch (23 cm) springform pan with cooking spray. Blot 5 pineapple rings dry with paper towels and arrange in a circle in the bottom of the pan. Place a cherry in the center of each pineapple ring.

② Place the remaining pineapple, reserved juice, ginger, cinnamon, and vanilla in a blender or food processor. Blend until smooth.

③ In a large heatproof bowl, beat egg yolks and brown sugar with an electric mixer on medium speed until thick and fluffy. Beat in the pineapple purée.

④ Bring 1 inch (2.5 cm) of water to a slow simmer in a large saucepan. Place the bowl of pineapple mixture over the simmering water (do not let bottom of bowl touch water). Beat on medium speed until thick, doubled in volume, and an instant-read thermometer registers 160°F (71°C). Carefully remove from the heat and continue beating on medium speed until room temperature. Set aside.

⑤ Clean and dry the beaters. In a second large bowl, beat egg whites, granulated sugar, and cream of tartar on medium speed until foamy. Set the bowl of egg whites over simmering water and beat on medium speed until the mixture is glossy and thick, about 3½ minutes. Increase the speed to high and continue beating until stiff and glossy, about 3½ minutes more or until egg whites reach 160°F (71°C). Remove from heat and beat on medium speed until room temperature. Whisk the meringue into the reserved pineapple mixture until smooth.

⑥ Clean and dry the beaters. In a medium bowl, beat cream with an electric mixer on high speed until soft peaks form. Fold the whipped cream into the batter. Pour the batter over the pineapple slices in the pan.

⑦ Cut angel food cake into slices and lay the slices over the batter covering the top. Cover with plastic wrap and freeze for at least 8 hours or up to 3 weeks.

YIELD: ONE 9-INCH (23 CM) CAKE, OR 10 SERVINGS

 **TO SERVE**

Let cake sit at room temperature for 10 to 15 minutes. Run a knife around the edges. Invert the pan onto a serving plate; gently tap to loosen the cake. Remove the pan sides and then carefully remove the pan bottom. If the bottom does not release easily, place a towel soaked in hot water on it for a minute and then try again.

> AMOUNT PER SERVING: Calories 212.81; Total Fat 6.17 g; Cholesterol 79.75 mg; Sodium 209.22 mg; Potassium 181.12 mg; Total Carbohydrates 36.21 g; Fiber 1.27 g; Sugar 21.39 g; Protein 4.57 g

# ACKNOWLEDGMENTS

My second cookbook, *Make-Ahead Meals Made Healthy*, could not have come to its flavorful fruition without the inspiration, support, opportunities, and love given to me by God and an extraordinary group of people.

My first thanks go to Will Kiester and Amanda Waddell of Fair Winds Press for giving me the grand opportunity of bringing the concept of a health-focused fix-and-freeze cookbook to life. I also thank Betsy Gammons, project manager, at Quayside Publishing Group for her keen eye for detail and gentle nudges to stay focused.

The most heartwarming thank you goes to my three-year-old son Tanner, who, at such a young age, is an eager and adventurous eater and a pint-size sous chef in his own right. Knowing that most of my recipes will be "quality-tested" by him furthers my tendency to make all of my meals with love.

Of course, I owe a never-ending thank you to the members of my family who have nourished me from the field and from the table, inspired my recipes, gifted me with countless kitchen gifts, and hungrily—and with sincerely deep appreciation—welcomed my meals. (I wish I could have sit-down meals with you all every day.)

A long-standing thank you goes to the many wonderful people I have worked with during the past nine years at sheknows.com. I appreciate the breadth of writing and editing opportunities you've given me.

I thank all of my friends who have shared recipes, meals, successful cooking stories, comical kitchen disasters, and cookbooks with me.

I give great thanks to God for his grace and for my family at Calvary Chapel Bozeman.

*"Whether you eat or drink, or whatever you do, do all to the glory of God."*

—Corinthians 10:31

# ABOUT THE AUTHOR

**MICHELE BORBOA, M.S.**, has been creating and cooking her own healthy freezer meals for more than twenty years, having gained her "make-ahead" start as a college student and long-distance runner in need of well-balanced, nutritious meals that could be prepared in no time. Today, as a mother, food columnist, and health and wellness expert, she often teaches others about the magic of make-ahead meals for fueling busy families right.

Michele is the author of the cookbook, *The Fitness Kitchen*, and holds a master's degree in exercise science and health promotion from California Polytechnic State University in San Luis Obispo, California. She is a food columnist at www.chefmom.com and channel editor at www.sheknows.com and has also been a personal chef for more than five years, specializing in healthy, practical meals. She lives with her family in Bozeman, Montana.

# INDEX